Second
UPDATED
Edition

Curbside Consultation in Retina

49 Clinical Questions

Curbside Consultation in Ophthalmology
Series

SERIES EDITOR, DAVID F. CHANG, MD

Curbside Consultation in Retina

49 Clinical Questions

Second UPDATED Edition

EDITED BY

Sharon Fekrat, MD, FACS

Professor, Ophthalmology
Associate Professor, Surgery
Director, Vitreoretinal Surgery Fellowship
Duke University School of Medicine
Associate Chief of Staff
Durham Veterans Affairs Medical Center
Durham, North Carolina

ASSOCIATE EDITORS

Akshay S. Thomas, MD, MS

Tennessee Retina
Nashville, Tennessee

Dilraj S. Grewal, MD

Associate Professor, Ophthalmology
Duke University School of Medicine
Durham, North Carolina

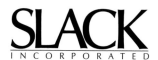

SLACK
INCORPORATED

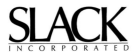

SLACK Incorporated
6900 Grove Road
Thorofare, NJ 08086 USA
856-848-1000   Fax: 856-848-6091
www.Healio.com/books
© 2019 by SLACK Incorporated

Senior Vice President: Stephanie Arasim Portnoy
Vice President, Editorial: Jennifer Kilpatrick
Vice President, Marketing: Michelle Gatt
Acquisitions Editor: Tony Schiavo
Managing Editor: Allegra Tiver
Creative Director: Thomas Cavallaro
Cover Artist: Katherine Christie
Project Editor: Emily Densten

The procedures and practices described in this publication should be implemented in a manner consistent with the professional standards set for the circumstances that apply in each specific situation. Every effort has been made to confirm the accuracy of the information presented and to correctly relate generally accepted practices. The authors, editors, and publisher cannot accept responsibility for errors or exclusions or for the outcome of the material presented herein. There is no expressed or implied warranty of this book or information imparted by it. Care has been taken to ensure that drug selection and dosages are in accordance with currently accepted/recommended practice. Off-label uses of drugs may be discussed. Due to continuing research, changes in government policy and regulations, and various effects of drug reactions and interactions, it is recommended that the reader carefully review all materials and literature provided for each drug, especially those that are new or not frequently used. Some drugs or devices in this publication have clearance for use in a restricted research setting by the Food and Drug and Administration or FDA. Each professional should determine the FDA status of any drug or device prior to use in their practice.

None of the information contained herein is intended for use in a court of law.

Any review or mention of specific companies or products is not intended as an endorsement by the author or publisher.

SLACK Incorporated uses a review process to evaluate submitted material. Prior to publication, educators or clinicians provide important feedback on the content that we publish. We welcome feedback on this work.

Library of Congress Cataloging-in-Publication Data

Names: Fekrat, Sharon, editor. | Thomas, Akshay S., editor. | Grewal, Dilraj
   S., editor.
Title: Curbside consultation in retina : 49 clinical questions / edited by
   Sharon Fekrat ; associate editors, Akshay S. Thomas, Dilraj S. Grewal.
Description: Second edition. | Thorofare, NJ : Slack Incorporated, [2019] |
   Series: Curbside consultation in ophthalmology series | Includes
   bibliographical references and index.
Identifiers: LCCN 2018029449 (print) | LCCN 2018030036 (ebook) | ISBN
   9781630914516 (epub) | ISBN 9781630914523 (web) | ISBN 9781630914509 (pbk.)
Subjects: | MESH: Retinal Diseases--diagnosis | Retinal Diseases--therapy
Classification: LCC RE551 (ebook) | LCC RE551 (print) | NLM WW 270 | DDC
   617.7/35--dc23
LC record available at https://lccn.loc.gov/2018029449

Printed in the United States of America.

Last digit is print number: 10   9   8   7   6   5   4   3   2   1

Dedication

We would like to dedicate this book to all individuals with retinal disease all over the world and all of those caring for them. We hope that this endeavor will facilitate the management of the retina conditions of millions.

Contents

Acknowledgments

We would like to acknowledge Darius Moshfeghi, MD and Dean Eliott, MD for their hard work on, and significant contributions to, the first edition of *Curbside Consultation in Retina* as Associate Editors. Their dedication to the first edition made it an excellent addition to medical bookshelves that has helped many patients around the world. Thank you!

About the Editor

Sharon Fekrat, MD, FACS is a vitreoretinal surgeon at the Duke University Eye Center, Professor of Ophthalmology and Associate Professor of Surgery at the Duke University School of Medicine, and Associate Chief of Staff at Duke's Veterans Affairs affiliate, the Durham Veterans Affairs Medical Center, where she previously held positions as Chief of Ophthalmology and Interim Chief of Surgery. She has co-authored over 120 peer-reviewed articles and over 40 book chapters, holds 2 surgical instrument patents, has received 2 American Society of Retina Specialists Rhett-Buckler Awards for surgical video, is on the editorial board of 6 professional journals, and has served as site principal investigator for numerous multicenter clinical trials. She is co-editor of Duke Eye Center's *All About Your Eyes* book for the lay public. Dr. Fekrat has been selected by her peers as one of Best Doctors each year for over a decade, was chosen as one of the top 150 leading retina innovators in the United States by *Ocular Surgery News*, and is past president of the North Carolina Society of Eye Physicians and Surgeons. She is Director of the Duke Vitreoretinal Surgery Fellowship and of Ophthalmology Faculty Mentoring and Career Development.

About the Associate Editors

Akshay S. Thomas, MD, MS is a Vitreoretinal Surgeon and Uveitis Specialist at Tennessee Retina. He has co-authored numerous peer-reviewed articles and book chapters, has served as an associate editor for the photoessay section of *Retina*, and was one of the recipients of the 2017 Ronald G. Michels Fellowship Award.

Dilraj S. Grewal, MD is an Associate Professor of Ophthalmology at Duke University, and is on the Vitreoretinal and Uveitis Service at the Duke University Eye Center. He also serves as Director of Grading at the Duke Reading Center. He has co-authored over 90 peer-reviewed publications and over 100 meeting abstracts. He serves as site principal investigator for several retina and uveitis clinical trials. Dr. Grewal has been recognized by the American Society of Retinal Specialists with the Honor Award and Rhett-Buckler Award and by the American Academy of Ophthalmology with the Achievement Award and multiple Best of Show awards.

Contributing Authors

Jackson Abou Chehade, MD (Question 37)
Post-Doctoral Research Fellow
Department of Ophthalmology
Mayo Clinic
Rochester, Minnesota

Ron A. Adelman, MD, MPH, MBA, FARVO (Question 40)
Professor of Ophthalmology and Visual Science
Director of the Retina and Macula Center
Yale University School of Medicine
New Haven, Connecticut

A. Yasin Alibhai, MD (Question 13)
New England Eye Center
Tufts Medical Center
Boston, Massachusetts

Michael T. Andreoli, MD (Question 33)
Wheaton Eye Clinic
Wheaton, Illinois

Sophie J. Bakri, MD (Question 11)
Mayo Clinic
Rochester, Minnesota

Alexander Barash, MD (Question 45)
New York Eye and Ear Infirmary
Mount Sinai Hospital
New York, New York

Caroline R. Baumal, MD (Question 44)
Associate Professor
Department Vitreoretinal Surgery
New England Eye Center
Department of Ophthalmology
Tufts University School of Medicine
Boston, Massachusetts

Daniel G. Cherfan, MD (Question 25)
Cole Eye Institute
Cleveland Clinic
Cleveland, Ohio

Michael N. Cohen, MD (Question 44)
Vitreoretinal Fellow
Department Vitreoretinal Surgery
New England Eye Center
Department of Ophthalmology
Tufts University School of Medicine
Boston, Massachusetts

Daniel Connors, MD (Question 27)
The Retina Institute
St. Louis, Missouri

Felipe F. Conti, MD (Question 30)
Cole Eye Institute
Center for Ophthalmic Bioinformatics
Cleveland Clinic
Cleveland, Ohio
Federal University of São Paulo
São Paulo, Brazil

Alessa Crossan, MD (Question 46)
Virginia Retina Center
Warrenton, Virginia

Cathy DiBernardo, CDOS (Question 7)
Duke Eye Center
University of North Carolina
Durham, North Carolina

Diana V. Do, MD (Question 4)
Professor of Ophthalmology
Byers Eye Institute
Stanford University School of Medicine
Palo Alto, California

Bernard H. Doft, MD (Question 19)
Retina Vitreous Consultants
University of Pittsburgh Medical Center
University of Pittsburgh School of Medicine
Pittsburgh, Pennsylvania

Mallika Doss, MD (Question 41)
University of Pittsburgh Medical Center
   Eye Center
Pittsburgh, Pennsylvania

Kimberly A. Drenser, MD, PhD (Question 49)
Associated Retinal Consultants
William Beaumont School of Medicine
Oakland University
Royal Oak, Michigan

Justis P. Ehlers, MD (Question 24)
Cole Eye Institute
Cleveland Clinic
Cleveland, Ohio

Dean Eliott, MD (Question 1)
Stelios Evangelos Gragoudas Associate
    Professor of Ophthalmology
Harvard Medical School
Associate Director, Retina Service
Massachusetts Eye and Ear Infirmary
Boston, Massachusetts

Nicholas Farber, MD (Question 18)
Vitreoretinal Surgeon
Southern Vitreoretinal Associates
Tallahassee, Florida

Amani A. Fawzi, MD (Question 23)
Department of Ophthalmology
Feinberg School of Medicine
Northwestern University
Chicago, Illinois

Avni P. Finn, MD, MBA (Question 34)
Northern California Retina Vitreous Associates
Mountain View, California

Harry W. Flynn, Jr., MD (Questions 14 and 43)
Department of Ophthalmology
Bascom Palmer Eye Institute
University of Miami
Miller School of Medicine
Miami, Florida

*Jose Mauricio Botto Garcia, MD, MSc
    (Question 5)*
Bascom Palmer Eye Institute
University of Miami
Miller School of Medicine
Miami, Florida

Seema Garg, MD, PhD (Question 17)
Associate Professor of Ophthalmology
University of North Carolina
Durham, North Carolina

Karen M. Gehrs, MD (Question 15)
Clinical Professor
University of Iowa
Iowa City, Iowa

*Ronald C. Gentile, MD, FACS, FASRS
    (Question 45)*
New York Eye and Ear Infirmary
Mount Sinai Hospital
New York, New York

Marina Gilca, MD (Questions 12 and 22)
Retina Consultants LTD
Fargo, North Dakota

Brian E. Goldhagen, MD (Question 48)
Assistant Professor of Clinical Ophthalmology
Bascom Palmer Eye Institute
University of Miami
Miller School of Medicine
Miami Veterans Affairs Healthcare System
Miami, Florida

Margaret A. Greven, MD (Question 4)
Assistant Professor of Ophthalmology
Wake Forest University School of Medicine
Winston-Salem, North Carolina

Paul Hahn, MD, PhD (Question 39)
Associate
NJRetina
Teaneck, New Jersey

Andrew M. Hendrick, MD (Question 9)
Emory University
Atlanta, Georgia

Odette Margit Houghton, MD (Question 18)
Senior Associate Consultant
Department of Ophthalmology
Mayo Clinic
Scottsdale, Arizona

Thomas Hwang, MD (Question 31)
Casey Eye Institute
Department of Ophthalmology
Oregon Health and Science University
Portland, Oregon

Alessandro Iannaccone, MD, MS, FARVO
(Question 38)
Professor of Ophthalmology
Director
Center for Retinal Degenerations and
   Ophthalmic Genetic Diseases
Duke Eye Center
Duke University School of Medicine
Durham, North Carolina

Raymond Iezzi, MD, MS (Question 37)
Department of Ophthalmology
Mayo Clinic
Rochester, Minnesota

Michael S. Ip, MD (Question 9)
David Geffen School of Medicine
University of California, Los Angeles
Doheny Eye Institute
Los Angeles, California

Yali Jia, PhD (Question 31)
Casey Eye Institute
Department of Ophthalmology
Oregon Health and Science University
Portland, Oregon

Scott Ketner, MD (Question 40)
Yale Eye Center
New Haven, Connecticut

Judy E. Kim, MD (Question 46)
Medical College of Wisconsin
Milwaukee, Wisconsin

Ryan S. Kim, BA (Question 21)
McGovern Medical School
University of Texas Health Science Center
Retina Consultants of Houston
Houston, Texas

Todd R. Klesert, MD, PhD (Question 8)
Vitreoretinal Associates of Washington
Bellevue, Washington

Linda A. Lam, MD, MBA (Question 47)
Associate Professor
USC Roski Eye Institute
USC Keck School of Medicine
Los Angeles, California

Jeremy A. Lavine, MD, PhD (Question 24)
Cole Eye Institute
Cleveland Clinic
Cleveland, Ohio

Phoebe Lin, MD, PhD (Question 35)
Assistant Professor of Ophthalmology
Casey Eye Institute
Oregon Health and Science University
Portland, Oregon

T. Y. Alvin Liu, MD (Question 2)
Wilmer Eye Institute
Johns Hopkins School of Medicine
Baltimore, Maryland

Tamer H. Mahmoud, MD, PhD (Question 34)
Professor of Ophthalmology
Oakland University William Beaumont
   School of Medicine
Associated Retinal Consultants
Royal Oak, Michigan

Joseph N. Martel, MD (Question 41)
Assistant Professor of Ophthalmology
University of Pittsburgh
Vitreoretinal Surgery and Diseases
University of Pittsburgh Medical Center
Pittsburgh, Pennsylvania

Pauline T. Merrill, MD (Question 22)
Illinois Retina Associates
Assistant Professor of Ophthalmology
Section Director, Uveitis and
   Ocular Inflammation
Rush University Medical Center
Chicago, Illinois

Catherine B. Meyerle, MD (Question 2)
Assistant Professor of Ophthalmology
Wilmer Eye Institute
Johns Hopkins School of Medicine
Baltimore, Maryland

William F. Mieler, MD (Question 33)
Cless Family Professor and Vice-Chairman
Director of Vitreoretinal Fellowship Training
Department of Ophthalmology and
   Visual Sciences
University of Illinois at Chicago
Chicago, Illinois

Prithvi Mruthyunjaya, MD, MHS
   (Question 20)
Associate Professor of Ophthalmology
Ocular Oncology and Vitreoretinal Surgery
Byers Eye Institute
Stanford University
Palo Alto, California

Lisa C. Olmos de Koo, MD, MBA (Question 32)
Associate Professor of Ophthalmology
Program Director
Vitreoretinal Surgery Fellowship
University of Washington Eye Institute
Seattle, Washington

Kaivon Pakzad-Vaezi, MD (Question 3)
Department of Ophthalmology and
   Visual Sciences
Faculty of Medicine
University of British Columbia
Vancouver, British Columbia, Canada

Amar Patel, MD (Question 36)
The Permanente Medical Group
Oakland, California

Kathryn L. Pepple, MD, PhD (Question 3)
Assistant Professor
University of Washington Eye Institute
Seattle, Washington

Sean M. Platt, MD (Question 11)
Mayo Clinic
Rochester, Minnesota

Matthew A. Powers, MD, MBA (Question 20)
Byers Eye Institute
Stanford University
Palo Alto, California

Franco M. Recchia, MD (Question 42)
Tennessee Retina, PC
Nashville, Tennessee

Nidhi Relhan Batra, MD (Question 43)
Department of Ophthalmology
Bascom Palmer Eye Institute
University of Miami
Miller School of Medicine
Miami, Florida

Kourous A. Rezaei, MD (Question 12)
Senior Partner
Director of Vitreoretinal Fellowship
Illinois Retina Associates
Associate Professor
Rush University Medical Center
Chicago, Illinois

Philipp Roberts, MD, PhD (Question 23)
Department of Ophthalmology and
   Optometry
Medical University of Vienna
Vienna, Austria

Philip J. Rosenfeld, MD, PhD (Question 5)
Bascom Palmer Eye Institute
University of Miami
Miller School of Medicine
Miami, Florida

SriniVas R. Sadda, MD (Question 28)
President and CSO
Stephen J. Ryan-Arnold and Mabel Beckman
   Endowed Chair
Professor of Ophthalmology
Doheny Eye Institute
University of California, Los Angeles
Los Angeles, California

Amy C. Schefler, MD (Question 21)
Retina Consultants of Houston
Blanton Eye Institute
Houston Methodist Hospital
Houston, Texas

Stephen G. Schwartz, MD, MBA (Question 14)
Department of Ophthalmology
Bascom Palmer Eye Institute
University of Miami
Miller School of Medicine
Miami, Florida

Steven D. Schwartz, MD (Question 6)
Stein Eye Institute
University of California, Los Angeles
Los Angeles, California

Ingrid U. Scott, MD, MPH (Question 14)
Jack and Nancy Turner Professor of
 Ophthalmology
Professor of Public Health Sciences
Associate Director of Ophthalmology
 Residency Program
Departments of Ophthalmology and Public
 Health Sciences
Penn State College of Medicine
Hershey, Pennsylvania

Michael I. Seider, MD (Question 36)
The Permanente Medical Group
San Francisco and Oakland, California
University of California, San Francisco
California Pacific Medical Group
San Francisco, California

Gaurav K. Shah, MD (Question 27)
The Retina Institute
St. Louis, Missouri

Sumit Sharma, MD (Question 25)
Assistant Professor of Ophthalmology
Cole Eye Institute
Cleveland Clinic
Cleveland, Ohio

Fabiana Q. Silva, MD (Question 30)
Cleveland Clinic Foundation
Cleveland, Ohio

Rishi P. Singh, MD (Question 30)
Staff Physician
Cole Eye Institute
Cleveland Clinic
Associate Professor of Ophthalmology
Lerner College of Medicine
Case Western Reserve University
Cleveland, Ohio

Richard F. Spaide, MD (Question 10)
Vitreous, Retina, Macula Consultants of
 New York
New York, New York

Sunil K. Srivastava, MD (Question 16)
Cleveland Clinic
Cleveland, Ohio

James A. Stefater, MD, PhD (Question 1)
Retina Fellow
Massachusetts Eye and Ear Infirmary
Harvard Medical School
Boston, Massachusetts

Arthi Venkat, MD (Question 16)
Cole Eye Institute
Cleveland Clinic
Cleveland, Ohio

Elizabeth Verner-Cole, MD (Question 35)
Associate
EyeHealth Northwest
Clinical Instructor
Oregon Health and Science University
Portland, Oregon

Nadia K. Waheed, MD, MPH (Question 13)
Tufts Medical Center
Tufts University School of Medicine
Boston Image Reading Center
Boston, Massachusetts

Scott D. Walter, MD, MSc (Question 29)
Associate
Retina Consultants, PC
Attending Physician
Hartford Hospital and Hartford Health Care
 Cancer Institute
Hartford, Connecticut

Charles C. Wykoff, MD, PhD (Question 43)
Retina Consultants of Houston
Blanton Eye Institute
Houston Methodist Hospital
Weill Cornell Medical College
Houston, Texas

Glenn Yiu, MD, PhD (Question 26)
Associate Professor
Department of Ophthalmology and
 Vision Science
University of California, Davis
Sacramento, California

Yoshihiro Yonekawa, MD (Question 49)
Massachusetts Eye and Ear Infirmary
Boston Children's Hospital
Harvard Medical School
Boston, Massachusetts

Preface

Are you seeking brief, evidence-based advice for the daily examination of patients? Are you looking for concise, practical answers to those questions that are often left unanswered by traditional references on the retina? The second edition of *Curbside Consultation in Retina: 49 Clinical Questions* provides quick and direct answers to questions most commonly posed during a "curbside consultation" between experienced clinicians. We have designed this unique reference so that it offers expert advice, preferences, and opinions on a variety of clinical questions commonly associated with different vitreoretinal clinical scenarios. The unique question-and-answer format provides quick access to current information related to the retina with the simplicity of a conversation between 2 colleagues. Images and references are included to enhance the text and to illustrate clinical diagnoses as well as ideas within the text. *Curbside Consultation in Retina: 49 Clinical Questions* provides information basic enough for residents while also incorporating expert pearls that even high-volume ophthalmologists and specialists will appreciate. Optometrists, ophthalmologists, ophthalmologists-in-training, and even retina specialists will benefit from the casual, user-friendly format and expert advice.

Foreword

Curbside consultations, either in person or via telephone, persist as an efficient means of obtaining sage advice in the daily practice of medicine. Enabling the transfer of information from a trusted colleague to the physician who is caring for the patient, curbside consultations persist because of their high intrinsic value. So too, Fekrat and colleagues' *Curbside Consultation in Retina* has proven its value and emerges updated, 8 year later, as a second edition. Once again, the erudite editors and co-authors parlay pearls in the management of retinal conditions typically found in a retinal practice. Questions posed are illustrative of scenarios arising daily in the care of retina patients. Answers are written in a style evocative of a conversation one would have with an expert in the field. Pragmatic advice not only jostles the reader's memory about the condition but also serves as a springboard from which to launch management.

This second edition still encompasses 49 clinical questions. However, over half of the curbside questions tackle new scenarios, technologies, and techniques relevant to today's practice. The editors were indeed not reticent in posing tantalizing and relevant questions to the featured experts. This second edition also updates salient questions from the first edition. Several chapters condense the information in tabular format that helps the reader readily digest and assimilate the information. Thus, the new compendium provides a wealth of information, presented efficiently and expertly, from sage colleagues to the reader. I very much enjoyed being a contributor to the first edition. Now, I am honored to extol this second edition. I am delighted that *Curbside Consultation in Retina* once again serves as a link between sage and vetted advice from a trusted colleague to the physician managing a patient in his or her office. Enjoy your curbside consults!

Jennifer I. Lim, MD, FARVO
Marion H. Schenk Esq. Chair in Ophthalmology for Research in the Aging Eye
Professor of Ophthalmology
Director of Retina
University of Illinois at Chicago
Illinois Eye and Ear Infirmary
Chicago, Illinois

Introduction

This book was put together just for you. Yup, just for you. Everything you wanted to know about 49 commonly asked retina questions in an easy format—just as if you called a retina colleague on the phone and said "What is hemorrhagic occlusive vasculitis and why do I need to know about it?" or "What is the easiest way to do a good B-scan?" or even better, "Why would I want to look at choroidal thickness on optical coherence tomography?" *Curbside Consultation in Retina* is exactly what it says it is: curbside consults for our colleagues—those in medical school, ophthalmology residency training, subspecialty fellowship training, optometry, ophthalmology, and even for retina specialists themselves.

As co-editors of *Curbside Consultation in Retina*, Akshay, Dilraj, and I have carefully chosen the questions to cover as many likely common clinical scenarios that need answers on a day-to-day basis as possible. What is special about this book is that of the 49 questions, there are more than 49 different authors who have done their vitreoretinal training in different institutions and who practice across the United States. This book does not represent the clinical practice or opinion of just one institution or group. Many authors are well-known experts in the specific area that is covered by the particular answer they authored. *Curbside Consultation* not only provides clinical opinion regarding the answers to different day-to-day questions at your fingertips but also offers an appropriate depth, and then some, gained from a "curbside consult."

As we all know, *Curbside Consultation in Retina* is not intended to substitute for appropriate education, training, and in some cases, vitreoretinal consultation. Instead, we hope that it will provide sufficient information that is readily available to guide your decision making in the common clinical scenarios discussed herein and prompt an appropriate referral when needed.

Turn the pages, and let the book draw you in.

Sharon Fekrat, MD, FACS

WHAT IS HEMORRHAGIC OCCLUSIVE RETINAL VASCULITIS, AND WHY DO I NEED TO KNOW ABOUT IT?

James A. Stefater MD, PhD

Dean Eliott, MD

Hemorrhagic occlusive retinal vasculitis (HORV) is a rare but devastating complication that has been described following uncomplicated cataract surgery. The first report describes 2 patients who had seemingly uneventful cataract surgery in the first eye but developed bilateral, severe, ischemic retinal vasculitis in both eyes within days following cataract surgery performed on the second eye.[1] Both patients had bilateral, severe, irreversible visual loss. Despite an extensive ocular and systemic work-up, a definitive causative factor was not identified; however, the authors note that both patients had received intraoperative intracameral vancomycin for endophthalmitis prophylaxis and proposed that intraoperative vancomycin exposure was the cause of the subsequent reaction. As word spread of the clinical findings and potential association, 4 additional patients were reported (3 bilateral, 1 unilateral) and these patients also had intraoperative exposure to vancomycin.[2]

The differential diagnosis of HORV includes acute postoperative endophthalmitis, viral retinitis, medication toxicity, and central retinal vein occlusion or combined central retinal artery and vein occlusions Most of these conditions can be ruled out after obtaining a thorough history and performing a careful examination.

A joint task force composed of a group of members from the American Society of Retina Specialists and the American Society of Cataract and Refractive Surgeons was formed to collect additional cases and to investigate causality. The task force ultimately identified a total of 36 eyes from 23 patients who likely had vancomycin-induced HORV.[3] All patients in this report had received vancomycin, either as an intracameral injection, in the irrigation solution during cataract surgery, or as intravitreal injection for the treatment of presumed endophthalmitis. Most patients had undergone uneventful first-eye cataract surgery but presented within a few days after second-eye cataract surgery with acute onset of painless visual loss in both eyes. In some patients, the

Fekrat S, ed. *Curbside Consultation in Retina: 49 Clinical Questions, Second Edition.* (pp 1-3).
© 2019 SLACK Incorporated

condition developed in one eye after the first-eye cataract surgery, and then also developed in the second eye after second-eye cataract surgery, even when the second surgery was performed years later. In these cases, vancomycin was used in both cataract surgeries.

The clinical findings of HORV are variable but include minimal anterior segment inflammation and severe retinal findings. There is typically a normal cornea or mild corneal edema, minimal anterior chamber reaction, and no hypopyon. The vitreous is clear or has mild inflammation. The retinal findings are usually profound and demonstrate diffuse retinal ischemia with severe, widespread intraretinal hemorrhages associated with retinal vasculitis. A few cases, however, had minimal symptoms and mild retinal findings. The outcome for most of these patients is devastating. Of the 36 eyes in the joint task force series, 8 had visual acuity of no light perception and 23 eyes (66%) were worse than 20/200.[3] Over 50% of eyes went on to develop neovascular glaucoma.[3]

It is worth noting that the association with vancomycin is only correlative; however, all reported cases to date have included vancomycin administration in some form. All cataract surgeries were performed by experienced surgeons and no additional cases from the same surgeon or the same surgery center were reported. The potential mechanism remains unknown, but the authors proposed the most likely mechanism to be a Type III hypersensitivity reaction where the patient receives intraocular vancomycin once without clinical sequelae, followed by a robust bilateral hypersensitivity response upon sequential administration. The time course is not consistent with direct toxicity because there is a delay (on average of 8 days) between the second-eye cataract surgery and presentation. In the cases that occurred after unilateral surgery, some patients reported systemic exposure to vancomycin in the past. Of note, a systemic leukocytoclastic vasculitis (where antigen-antibody complexes deposit in vessel walls) has been reported to occur with systemic administration of vancomycin,[4] and HORV is presumed to occur via a similar mechanism. This proposed etiology raises the issue of whether aggressive management with immunosuppressive agents could play a therapeutic role. Importantly, in cases where early steroids were implemented, visual prognosis was generally better. According to the joint task force, the 3 eyes that received intravitreal corticosteroids had final visual outcomes of 20/40, 20/70, and hand motion. Early treatment with anti-vascular endothelial growth factor agents and early panretinal photocoagulation also appeared to result in better outcomes.

While causality cannot be definitively determined, and while the response is admittedly extremely rare (the vast majority of patients receive vancomycin without a similar response), the devastating nature of this condition should prompt careful consideration as to the necessity of prophylactic vancomycin during cataract surgery. The seminal study on antibiotic use during cataract surgery to prevent endophthalmitis had a profound impact on the practice patterns of surgeons in Europe.[5] In this study, the endophthalmitis rate decreased from 0.34% to 0.07% with the use of intracameral cefuroxime. Many US surgeons were skeptical of the results because of the high rate of endophthalmitis in the control group (0.34%). However, over the last 10 years, the trend among US cataract surgeons has begun to shift. In 2007, only 15% of cataract surgeons were using intraoperative prophylactic antibiotics, but in 2014, 36% of surgeons were using such therapy.[6] Of those surgeons, 15% were using vancomycin in the infusion solution and 22% were performing a direct intracameral injection of vancomycin. In total, 13% of all cataract surgeons in the United States in 2014 were using intraoperative vancomycin.[6] Out of the patients receiving antibiotic prophylaxis but not receiving vancomycin, the most common agent was moxifloxacin (33%) followed by a cephalosporin (26%).[6] Interestingly, there are no reports of HORV in patients who received moxifloxacin or cefuroxime.[3]

If cataract surgeons nonetheless choose to use vancomycin, and a patient presents to a retina specialist, making the correct diagnosis and distinguishing the clinical presentation of HORV from endophthalmitis is of critical importance. Some patients who presented with visual loss after cataract surgery were presumed to have mild endophthalmitis (no hypopyon) when they likely had HORV instead. These eyes received intravitreal vancomycin and had exceptionally poor outcomes.

In some of these eyes, fluorescein angiography documented retinal ischemia after the cataract surgery which worsened after the intravitreal vancomycin injection.

Summary

Ophthalmologists should suspect HORV when a patient develops visual loss after unilateral or bilateral cataract surgery along with the findings indicated previously. Retina specialists should inquire about the use of intraoperative vancomycin. It is critical to distinguish HORV from early endophthalmitis so that additional vancomycin is not administered in an eye with possible HORV. Early treatment with intravitreal, periocular, and/or systemic steroids as well as intravitreal anti-vascular endothelial growth factor agents and panretinal photocoagulation may offer some benefit. It is also important to remember that if HORV develops in one eye after unilateral cataract surgery, there is evidence that the second eye can undergo successful cataract surgery provided vancomycin is not used.

References

1. Nicholson LB, Kim BT, Jardon J, et al. Severe bilateral ischemic retinal vasculitis following cataract surgery. *Ophthalmic Surg Lasers Imaging Retina*. 2014;45(4):338-342.
2. Witkin AJ, Shah AR, Engstrom RE, et al. Postoperative hemorrhagic occlusive retinal vasculitis: expanding the clinical spectrum and possible association with vancomycin. *Ophthalmology*. 2015;122(7):1438-1451.
3. Witkin AJ, Chang DF, Jumper JM, et al. Vancomycin-associated hemorrhagic occlusive retinal vasculitis: clinical characteristics of 36 eyes. *Ophthalmology*. 2017;124(5):583-595.
4. Pongruangporn M, Ritchie DJ, Lu D, Marschall J. Vancomycin-associated leukocytoclastic vasculitis. *Case Rep Infect Dis*. 2011;2011:356370.
5. Endophthalmitis Study Group, European Society of Cataract & Refractive Surgeons. Prophylaxis of postoperative endophthalmitis following cataract surgery: results of the ESCRS multicenter study and identification of risk factors. *J Cataract Refract Surg*. 2007;33(6):978-988.
6. Chang DF, Braga-Mele R, Henderson BA, Mamalis N, Vasavada A; ASCRS Cataract Clinical Committee. Antibiotic prophylaxis of postoperative endophthalmitis after cataract surgery: results of the 2014 ASCRS member survey. *J Cataract Refract Surg*. 2015;41(6):1300-1305.

HOW DO I COUNSEL MY PATIENTS WITH DRY AGE-RELATED MACULAR DEGENERATION AND WHAT ABOUT VARIOUS VITAMIN SUPPLEMENTS?

T. Y. Alvin Liu, MD

Catherine B. Meyerle, MD

Let us first review the rationale and results of the original Age-Related Eye Disease Study (AREDS). Beginning in the early 1990s, several observational studies showed the protective association of increased antioxidant vitamin intake with decreased risk of age-related macular degeneration (AMD) development. AREDS, beginning in 2001 under National Eye Institute sponsorship, was designed to evaluate this suggested nutritional role in a prospective clinical trial. Specifically, AREDS was a 5-year randomized study of 4757 participants evaluating whether high-dose antioxidants and zinc could reduce progression of both AMD and age-related lens opacity. Participants were categorized according to drusen size. Small drusen were defined as less than 63 μm, intermediate drusen as 63 μm to 124 μm, and large drusen as greater than or equal to 125 μm. Patients were then randomized to oral supplementation of high-dose antioxidant vitamins and/or zinc. Final analysis demonstrated that 500 mg vitamin C, 400 IU vitamin E, 15 mg beta-carotene, and 80 mg zinc oxide (along with 2 mg cupric oxide to prevent copper-deficiency anemia) reduced the risk of advanced AMD, defined as neovascular AMD or geographic atrophy (GA) involving the fovea, by 25% in participants with intermediate AMD (extensive intermediate drusen and/or any large drusen) or with advanced AMD in one eye.[1]

A second trial known as AREDS2 further refined the antioxidant clinical trial data. The impetus for this randomized clinical trial of 4203 participants was dietary data obtained from the original AREDS participants and nutritional concerns regarding beta-carotene and zinc. During AREDS, all participants completed a food frequency questionnaire. Baseline intake of lutein/zeaxanthin and carotenoids found in dark green leafy vegetables, such as spinach, collard greens, and kale, was inversely associated with neovascular AMD, GA, and large or extensive

Fekrat S, ed. *Curbside Consultation in Retina: 49 Clinical Questions, Second Edition.* (pp 5-8).
© 2019 SLACK Incorporated

intermediate drusen.[2] This is noteworthy because macular pigment is composed primarily of lutein/zeaxanthin, and these carotenoids are postulated to protect the retina from oxidative stress. Lutein and zeaxanthin were not included in the original AREDS study because they were not readily available for manufacturing in a research formulation at that time. A second dietary factor that was significant was the baseline intake of omega-3 long-chain polyunsaturated fatty acids derived from fish. Higher fish consumption was inversely associated with neovascular AMD.[3] Based on these nutritional associations, AREDS2 enrollment began in 2006 to determine whether oral supplementation with macular xanthophylls (lutein 10 mg/day and zeaxanthin 2 mg/day) and/or omega-3 long-chain polyunsaturated fatty acids (docosahexaenoic acid [DHA] 350 mg/day and eicosapentaenoic acid [EPA] 650 mg/day, for a total of 1 g of fish oil/day) would decrease the risk of progression to advanced AMD as compared to the control group of those receiving the original AREDS formula. Given the increased risk of lung cancer with beta-carotene use among smokers and the fact that beta-carotene is not found within human ocular tissue unlike lutein/zeaxanthin, a secondary randomization in AREDS2 evaluated whether it would be worthwhile to remove beta-carotene from the AREDS2 formula. The final research question involved zinc. Although there was decreased mortality overall in the zinc group in AREDS, nutritional experts have been increasingly concerned about high-dose zinc usage. In addition to the increased genitourinary complications found in AREDS, zinc has been reported to have an adverse effect on cholesterol levels in other studies. Based on these concerns, the second randomization in AREDS2 investigated whether lowering zinc to 25 mg/day would be beneficial.

As the original AREDS study detected an overall low risk for early AMD cases converting to advanced disease, the AREDS2 study did not include early AMD cases and only enrolled patients with a higher risk of progression to advanced AMD: bilateral large drusen or large drusen in one eye and advanced AMD in the fellow eye. The results, published in 2013,[4] were as follows: The primary randomization showed that the addition of lutein + zeaxanthin, DHA + EPA or lutein + zeaxanthin + DHA + EPA to the original AREDS formulation, as compared to the original formulation alone, did not reduce the chance of progression to advanced AMD or vision loss. However, an exploratory, ad hoc, subgroup analysis showed that the addition of lutein and zeaxanthin was beneficial in patients with baseline low dietary intake of lutein and zeaxanthin (bottom quintile), so it may help those with a diet lacking in green leafy vegetables or other dietary sources of lutein. It is also interesting to note that the addition of omega-3 fatty acid (DHA and EPA) did not confer any benefits, which was in contrast to a previous study that showed higher fish consumption was inversely associated with neovascular AMD.[3] Perhaps, there is a biochemical difference between the omega-3 fatty acid in pill form and that found in traditional dietary intake; more studies are needed in this area. In the secondary randomization, it was shown that removing beta-carotene, reducing the zinc dosage, or removing beta-carotene plus reducing the zinc dosage also did not confer any additional benefits.

Now that we have reviewed the basic principles of the AREDS and AREDS2 studies, let us discuss how we apply these clinical trial results to our everyday practice. First, we believe both the original AREDS and AREDS2 formulae are equally efficacious for nonsmoking patients with intermediate or advanced AMD in one eye. However, if our patient with intermediate or advanced AMD in one eye smokes, we do not initiate the original antioxidant formula given the aforementioned risk of beta-carotene among smokers. As it is not known if a past smoking history in conjunction with beta-carotene puts patients at additional risk, we recommend AREDS2 for both current and prior smokers. Second, we do not recommend either AREDS formulation for patients with early AMD defined as multiple small drusen or rare intermediate drusen. These patients had a low rate of developing advanced AMD during AREDS (1.3% in 5 years), so antioxidant supplementation is not beneficial in such cases. Instead, we counsel these early AMD patients about the importance of regular dilated eye examinations and a healthy diet, including lots of fruits and vegetables. Third, for reasons discussed previously, we do not recommend antioxidant therapy for the offspring of affected individuals unless they personally meet the criteria for intermediate or advanced AMD in one eye. Fourth, when patients with bilateral advanced AMD inquire if they should take the original AREDS formula, we tell them that the study was designed to evaluate risk reduction for progressing to advanced AMD so there is no data to answer the question of whether these patients still benefit from the formulation or not. The long-term effects (10 years) of the original AREDS formula were published in 2013, showing that patients with intermediate or advanced AMD in one eye who were originally assigned to the AREDS formulation, as compared to the placebo group, continued to show statistically significant reduction in the development of moderate vision loss, advanced AMD, and neovascular AMD but not central GA. Also, patients with central GA have been shown to be at a high risk for developing neovascular AMD, as high as 40% over 10 years.[5] Hence, it is reasonable to extrapolate that patients with bilateral advanced AMD, in the form of central GA, may benefit from continuation of the AREDS formulation by potentially decreasing the chance of conversion to neovascular AMD that will further affect their vision. However, further research is needed for definitive answers in this bilaterally advanced patient group. Lastly, for patients already taking the original AREDS formulation, there is no definite contraindication for them to take additional over-the-counter vitamin supplements. The concentration of vitamins in typical over-the-counter supplements is much lower than that in the AREDS formulation and general multivitamins often contain additional nutritional supplementation that is not included in the AREDS formula. In fact, about 67% of AREDS participants chose to take Centrum along with the study medication and there was no definitive evidence that a higher rate of adverse events occurred in this group.[1]

While the AREDS antioxidant formula has had a major public health impact in terms of preventing advanced AMD, it can have side effects just like all medications. Fortunately, the adverse event rate is low. As mentioned previously, beta-carotene supplementation is contraindicated in smokers. Beta-carotene occasionally caused yellow discoloration of the skin in both smokers and nonsmokers, but this was of no health consequence. Also, patients randomized to zinc had an increase in genitourinary complications, such as urinary tract infection, prostate hyperplasia, and stress incontinence. However, an analysis of zinc vs no zinc found a statistically significant reduction in mortality in the zinc group (relative risk 0.73, 95% CI: 0.61 to 0.89), so, overall, the original AREDS formulation is safe. In AREDS2, addition of lutein and zeaxanthin to the original formula, as compared to the original formula alone, did not increase the rate of serious adverse events. More lung cancers were observed in the beta-carotene group as compared to the no–beta-carotene group, but 91% of participants who developed lung cancer were former smokers. Finally, there was no difference in the rates of reported gastrointestinal disorders and hospitalizations for genitourinary diseases between the high- and low-dose zinc groups.[4]

Some meta-analyses have warned of increased morbidity and mortality associated with vitamin therapy.[6,7] The methodology of these meta-analyses, however, is questionable. Some used flawed subgroup analysis to support their claims. Others focused on large beta-carotene trials that included smokers, thus creating a negative bias. Due to the low adverse event rate in AREDS, we feel that the original AREDS formula is safe in nonsmokers. Additionally, availability of AREDS2 now offers a formula that is safe for smokers as it contains lutein instead of beta-carotene. Both AREDS studies have had a significant impact on risk reduction for progression to advanced AMD, but further nutritional research is required to help those who already have bilateral advanced AMD.

References

1. Age-Related Eye Disease Study Research Group. A randomized, placebo-controlled, clinical trial of high-dose supplementation with vitamins C and E, beta carotene, and zinc for age-related macular degeneration and vision loss: AREDS report no. 8. *Arch Ophthalmol.* 2001;119(10):1417-1436.
2. SanGiovanni JP, Chew EY; Age-Related Eye Disease Study Research Group. The relationship of dietary carotenoid and vitamin A, E, and C intake with age-related macular degeneration in a case-control study: AREDS Report No. 22. *Arch Ophthalmol.* 2007;125(9):1225-1232.
3. SanGiovanni JP, Chew EY, Clemons TE, et al. The relationship of dietary lipid intake and age-related macular degeneration in a case-control study: AREDS Report No. 20. *Arch Ophthalmol.* 2007;125(5):671-679.
4. Age-Related Eye Disease Study 2 Research G. Lutein + zeaxanthin and omega-3 fatty acids for age-related macular degeneration: the Age-Related Eye Disease Study 2 (AREDS2) randomized clinical trial. *JAMA.* 2013;309(19):2005-2015.
5. Chew EY, Clemons TE, Agron E, et al. Long-term effects of vitamins C and E, beta-carotene, and zinc on age-related macular degeneration: AREDS report no. 35. *Ophthalmology.* 2013;120(8):1604-1611, e1604.
6. Bjelakovic G, Nikolova D, Gluud LL, Simonetti RG, Gluud C. Mortality in randomized trials of antioxidant supplements for primary and secondary prevention: systematic review and meta-analysis. *JAMA.* 2007;297(8):842-857.
7. Miller ER III, Pastor-Barriuso R, Dalal D, Riemersma RA, Appel LJ, Guallar E. Meta-analysis: high-dosage vitamin E supplementation may increase all-cause mortality. *Ann Intern Med.* 2005;142(1):37-46.

WHAT ARE THE AGE-RELATED MACULAR DEGENERATION LOOK-ALIKES? DO I TREAT THEM ANY DIFFERENTLY?

Kaivon Pakzad-Vaezi, MD
Kathryn L. Pepple, MD, PhD

The majority of clinical practice adheres to the classic medical aphorism, "When you hear hoof beats, think of horses not zebras." However, not every patient presenting with macular drusen, pigmentary changes, or areas of retinal pigment epithelium (RPE) atrophy carries the straightforward diagnosis of non-neovascular (or dry) age-related macular degeneration (AMD). Detecting zebras in the herd affords the clinician an opportunity to identify and treat systemic disease, neoplasia, or a genetic mutation with multigenerational implications.

Suspicion for an AMD look-alike should be spurred when typical signs of AMD are detected at an earlier age than expected or in association with specific clinical patterns. Variations in the typical signs (ie, drusen, pigmentary change, RPE atrophy) that should tip you off to an atypical case are listed in Table 3-1. When clinical suspicion for atypical AMD is high, increased attention should be paid to the clinical history, including age of presentation, initial fundus changes, the degree of visual acuity loss, and especially to subtle or pronounced nyctalopia. The review of systems should probe for problems with hearing, diabetes, renal disease, or skin problems. A history of current or prior steroid use should be elicited. The family history is also informative and will often identify relatives carrying a diagnosis of early onset AMD, unexplained visual loss and blindness, or occasionally nyctalopia. In some cases, examination of accompanying family members can be revealing. It is unusual for the diagnosis of an AMD mimic to be made solely with dilated fundus examination. Common ancillary tests including fundus photography, fundus autofluorescence (FAF), and optical coherence tomography (OCT) are complementary modalities used in developing the initial differential diagnosis. Ultimately, electroretinography (ERG) and/or electrooculograms (EOG) may be required in association with genetic testing to clarify the diagnosis.

Fekrat S, ed. *Curbside Consultation in Retina: 49 Clinical Questions, Second Edition.* (pp 9-17).
© 2019 SLACK Incorporated

Table 3-1

Approach to Atypical Non-Neovascular Age-Related Macular Degeneration

Sign	Suggestive Imaging Features	Diagnoses to Consider
1. Drusen		
a. Cuticular drusen	• OCT—prolate shape, sub-RPE material, sawtooth pattern • FAF—hypoautofluorescent • FA—"starry sky" hyperfluorescence	• AMD • MPGN Type II
b. Subretinal drusenoid deposits	• OCT—subretinal material • FAF—typically hypoautofluorescent, rarely hyperautofluorescent, peripheral scalloped hypoautofluorescence (*C1QTNF5*)	• *EFEMP1* • *TIMP3* • *C1QTNF5 (LORD)* • MPGN Type II • North Carolina macular dystrophy, Grades I and II
c. Macular flecks	• OCT—subretinal hyperreflective material, ellipsoid layer disruption • FAF—typically hyperautofluorescent, angioid streaks (*ABCC6*)	• *ABCA4* • *PRPH2* • MIDD • Myotonic dystrophy • Pseudoxanthoma elasticum (*ABCC6*)
d. Vitelliform lesions	• OCT—subretinal hyperreflective material • FAF—hyperautofluorescent	• Best macular dystrophy • Adult vitelliform macular dystrophy • Coalesced soft drusen • Rare: acute exudative vitelliform maculopathy • Rare: paraneoplastic vitelliform maculopathy

(continued)

Table 3-1 (continued)

Approach to Atypical Non-Neovascular Age-Related Macular Degeneration

Sign	Suggestive Imaging Features	Diagnoses to Consider
2. Pigmentary Change		
a. Nonspecific pigmentary changes	• OCT—variable outer retinal loss, subretinal hyperreflective material, pigment epithelial detachments, thickened choroid • FAF—mixed hyper/hypoautofluorescence, gravitational tracts	• Central serous chorioretinopathy • Pachychoroid pigment epitheliopathy
3. Geographic Atrophy		
a. Late-stage inherited dystrophies	• FAF—flecks (*ABCA4, PRPH2*), peripheral scalloped hypoautofluorescence (*C1QTNF5*), parafoveal atrophy (MIDD), crystals (Bietti)	• *ABCA4* • *PRPH2* • *C1QTNF5* • Best macular dystrophy • MIDD • Bietti retinal dystrophy
b. Inflammatory	• Color—serpiginoid pattern, multifocal pattern • FA—early hypofluorescence, late leak during active stages. Occasional edge staining in late stage. Staining of subretinal fibrosis.	• Macular serpiginous • Tuberculosis serpiginous-like choroiditis • APMPPE • Subretinal fibrosis
c. Miscellaneous		• Macular/congenital Toxoplasma gondii infection • North Carolina macular dystrophy, Grade III

FA=fluorescein angiography; MIDD=maternally inherited diabetes and deafness; MPGN=membranoproliferative glomerulonephritis; LORD=late-onset retinal degeneration; APMPPE=acute posterior multifocal placoid pigment epitheliopathy

While there is considerable overlap in fundus appearance of many of the AMD mimics with typical AMD, and while no single imaging test is diagnostic for any one condition, we find the following 2-step approach helpful in building a more focused differential diagnosis. The first step is to separate the differential based on the predominance of drusenoid and pigmentary changes vs RPE atrophic changes. We then use OCT and FAF to better characterize the changes as typical or atypical in appearance. Finally, in the case that clinical history and imaging support the concern for an atypical AMD case, more extensive testing with electrophysiology, targeted laboratory evaluation, and genetic testing is pursued.

How We Use Typical and Atypical Drusen to Direct Diagnostic Work-Up

We first characterize the drusen based on OCT and FAF appearance. The typical drusen of AMD include macular yellow-white, round-ovoid elevations of various sizes and number in the macula in people over 55 years of age.[1] OCT morphology can vary, but common AMD-related drusen demonstrate hyperreflective elevations at the level of the RPE with mixed FAF.[2] Small (< 63 μm) macular drusen in the absence of other findings are thought to reflect normal aging changes and do not require work-up or treatment.[3] Likewise, peripheral drusen are a common finding in the elderly and, in the absence of macular drusen, are not included in current AMD classifications.[3] It is also rare that they suggest pathology that requires additional evaluation.

Cuticular drusen (Figure 3-1) are associated most often with typical AMD, but they are also the most common drusen type associated with MPGN II.[2] They are identified by their prolate shape on OCT, "sawtooth" profile, and are hypoautofluorescent on FAF.[2] MPGN II is typically diagnosed between the ages of 5 to 15 years, with vision loss occurring as a late complication; however, in the correct clinical context, renal function tests and urinalysis should be considered as part of the evaluation of cuticular drusen in a young person.

Subretinal drusenoid deposits (SDD) (Figure 3-2) refer to hyperreflective material located between the retina and RPE instead of at or below the level of the RPE on OCT. They are often hypoautofluorescent, but occasionally may be hyperautofluorescent and, in these cases, are particularly suggestive of an inherited dystrophy.[2] They are occasionally present along with typical drusen in patients with AMD; however, a predominance of SDD suggests alternative diagnoses, such as an inherited retinal dystrophy or vitamin A deficiency. Vitamin A deficiency can produce anterior segment changes and ERG abnormalities and can be easily screened with a blood test. If confirmed, supplementation can produce dramatic recovery.[4] Taking a history of nyctalopia is particularly helpful in these cases. Examples of genetic dystrophies that cause SDD include dominant drusen (*EFEMP1*), Sorsby fundus dystrophy (*TIMP3*), MPGN II, North Carolina macular dystrophy (Grades I and II), pseudoxanthoma elasticum (*ABCC6*), and LORD (*C1QTNF5*).[2,5] Diagnostic clues include dominant inheritance (*EFEMP1, TIMP3, C1QTNF5*), early nyctalopia and ERG changes (*TIMP3, C1QTNF5*), aggressive choroidal neovascularization (CNV; *TIMP3*), angioid streaks (*ABCC6*), long anterior lens zonules and scalloped peripheral atrophic changes (*C1QTNF5*), and renal disease (MPGN II).

When the lesions look more like flecks on OCT and FAF, a new set of different diagnoses are prompted. Flecks are differentiated from drusen by the lack of uniform round-oval, dome-shaped appearance, the distribution, and the usually yellow/vitelliform appearance. While drusen tend to stain on FA, flecks demonstrate blockage from lipofuscin, or variable window defect if adjacent RPE has degenerated.[6] We find FAF to be the most helpful in not only demonstrating hyperautofluorescence of the flecks, but also to reveal more extensive fundus involvement than

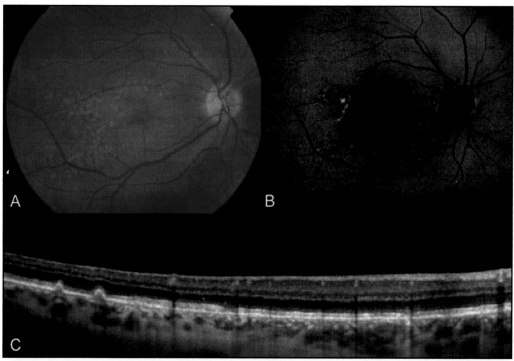

Figure 3-1. Cuticular drusen. (A) Numerous small and medium cuticular sub-RPE drusen are demonstrated. (B) They are predominantly hypoautofluorescent. (C) Prolate, sawtooth appearance. Note: these drusen are sub-RPE, while the drusen in Figure 3-2 are subretinal. (Reprinted with permission from Khan KN, Mahroo OA, Khan RS, et al. Differentiating drusen: Drusen and drusen-like appearances associated with ageing, age-related macular degeneration, inherited eye disease and other pathological processes. *Prog Retin Eye Res.* 2016;53:70-106.)

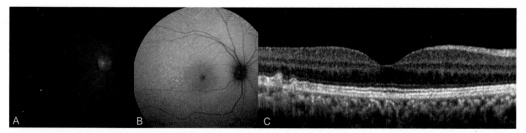

Figure 3-2. Dominant drusen (EFEMP1). (A) Foveal and extrafoveal drusen. (B) Drusen hyper-autofluorescence. (C) Subretinal location of drusenoid material on OCT.

appreciated clinically. Stargardt disease (fundus flavimaculatus, *ABCA4*-retinopathy) (Figure 3-3) is the prototype fleck dystrophy. It often presents in childhood with decreased central vision, although adult-onset cases are well-described.[7] An autosomal recessive inheritance pattern may be elicited, and we recommend baseline ERG for prognostication[8] as well as avoidance of high-dose vitamin A supplementation.[9] The classic dark choroid on FA is rare with modern fundus cameras, and, as such, we reserve FA solely to rule out CNV. Pattern dystrophy (Figure 3-4), which can also present with flecks and can be difficult to differentiate clinically from *ABCA4*-retinopathy, often presents in mid- or late-life as atypical AMD. Multiple patterns of vitelliform flecks have previously been described clinically.[6] In the era of molecular genetics, most of these are recognized as an autosomal dominant-inherited defect in *PRPH2*.[10] Many patients are asymptomatic and this

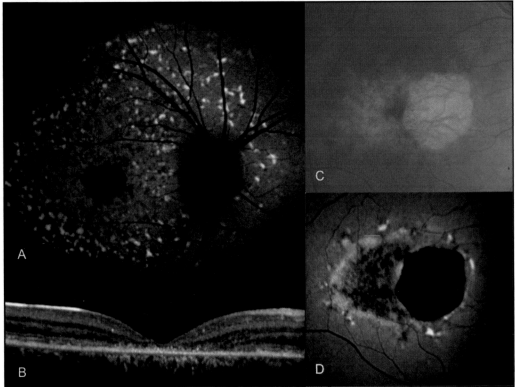

Figure 3-3. Stargardt disease (*ABCA4*-retinopathy). (A) FAF reveals hyperautofluorescence of flecks that are often difficult to visualize on clinical examination alone; in this case also demonstrating classic peripapillary sparing of flecks. (B) OCT shows outer retinal atrophy and small SDD. (C) A different patient with Stargardt demonstrating geographic atrophy. (D) Typical hyperautofluorescent flecks surrounding the area of atrophy provide a clue to the underlying diagnosis.

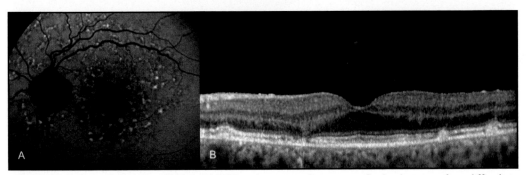

Figure 3-4. Pattern dystrophy (*PRPH2*). (A) Diffuse hyperautofluorescent flecks that are often difficult to fully appreciate on clinical examination. (B) Flecks corresponding to SDD on OCT.

may only be detected on routine ocular exam. Armed with a strong family history of AMD, they often present erroneously, taking Age-Related Eye Disease Study (AREDS) formulations. Clues for diagnosis include traditional patterns (ie, butterfly, reticular, multifocal, pulverulentus),[6] usually a paucity of drusen, and/or symmetric central vitelliform lesions that are hyperautofluorescent as in adult vitelliform macular dystrophy (AVMD). Symptomatically, these patients present for 2 main reasons: expanding RPE atrophy or CNV. Of note, a partially collapsed vitelliform lesion can mimic subretinal fluid; clues to rule out CNV can be appreciated on FA, indocyanine green,

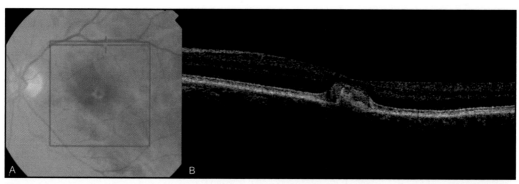

Figure 3-5. AVMD. (A) Foveal vitelliform lesion with central pigmentation, mimicking typical drusen. (B) Subretinal vitelliform material not consistent with typical drusen on OCT.

previous OCT, or a typical vitelliform lesion in the other eye. Finally, one should remember that flecks can accompany such systemic conditions as MIDD, pseudoxanthoma elasticum (*ABCC6*), Alport syndrome, and myotonic dystrophy.[6] Appropriate questioning and examination should therefore be prompted.

Finally, the appearance of vitelliform lesions on OCT and FAF are quite typical and suggest other non–AMD diagnoses. Vitelliform lesions refer to yellow fundus lesions that usually correspond to subretinal (not sub-RPE) hyperreflective material on OCT, and hyperautofluorescent lesions on FAF. While confluent soft drusen can mimic such an appearance, these are usually sub-RPE on OCT and not hyperautofluorescent to the same degree. Best Disease (*BEST1*) is the prototype vitelliform macular dystrophy, but is easily differentiated with its clinical appearance, early age of onset, dominant family history, and EOG findings. As alluded to previously, the AVMD (Figure 3-5) variant of *PRPH2*-retinopathy is more often mistaken for either dry or wet AMD due to its age of presentation. These patients occasionally present after having received multiple anti-vascular endothelial growth factor (anti-VEGF) injections without response. They are often minimally symptomatic until either the natural collapse of the vitelliform lesions with subsequent RPE atrophy (Figure 3-6) or the development of CNV. Prior to this, however, they may be referred to the retina specialist with bilateral, symmetric hyperautofluorescent vitelliform lesions. The recognition of this dystrophy will save the patient costly medication and intravitreal injections, replaced by daily Amsler grid monitoring. Finally, the appearance of multiple vitelliform lesions, typically acutely, should prompt the consideration of the rare acute exudative polymorphous vitelliform maculopathy and paraneoplastic vitelliform retinopathy, with the exclusion of cutaneous and uveal malignant melanoma required in the latter.[11,12]

Pigmentary changes associated with chronic and/or resolved central serous chorioretinopathy and pachychoroid pigment epitheliopathy deserve mention. These can be mistaken for drusen and/or pigmentary abnormalities, but usually offer such differentiating features as asymmetry, reduced fundus tessellation, relatively increased choroidal thickness compared to AMD, and gravitational fluid tracts on FAF.[13,14]

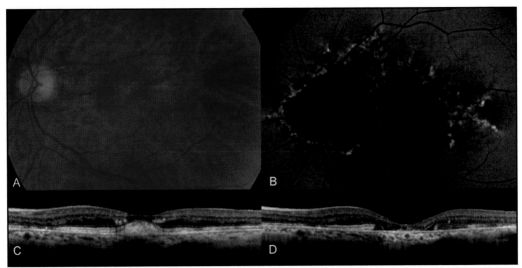

Figure 3-6. Pattern dystrophy, in this case due to MIDD. (A) Drusenoid and fleck-like lesions, the full extent of which is difficult to appreciate. (B) Hyperautofluorescent flecks are more apparent on autofluorescence. (C) Corresponding OCT shows a central vitelliform lesion in this patient who is largely asymptomatic. (D) However, 3 years later, she returned with reduced central vision due to collapse of the vitelliform lesion with associated outer retinal and RPE atrophy.

How We Use Atypical Geographic Atrophy to Direct Diagnostic Work-Up

The late stage of many of the previously mentioned inherited macular/retinal dystrophies, including the addition of Bietti retinal dystrophy, demonstrate variable degrees of RPE atrophy (see Figure 3-3). For us, non–AMD diagnoses are prompted when there is a lack of drusen, earlier age of onset, nyctalopia, suggestive family history, and previous imaging and electrodiagnostics. Specific features include the peripheral retinal degeneration of LORD, the crystals in Bietti dystrophy, angioid streaks in pseudoxanthoma elasticum, and the auditory changes along with the kidney-shaped perifoveal RPE atrophy occasionally seen in MIDD.

Inflammatory mimics of geographic atrophy should be kept in mind. Conditions like serpiginous choroiditis and APMPPE leave a legacy of RPE atrophy. Typical serpiginous, however, extends from a peripapillary location, is asymmetrically bilateral, and often has evidence of current or previous vitreous inflammation. Alternatively, atypical serpiginous, such as the macular variant, does not extend from the optic nerve; in this case, the lack of drusen, evidence of prior inflammation, and the disease course are helpful. After infectious causes are ruled out (particularly tuberculosis), we monitor these patients for inflammatory disease recurrence and the development of CNV. Finally, an exuberant postinflammatory subretinal fibrotic response can occur in some uveitic conditions, occasionally mimicking the disciform scar of AMD. Again, historical investigation and signs of previous inflammatory activity can assist in differentiation.

Using this approach, when we classify an atypical AMD as one of the previously mentioned diagnoses, our treatment recommendations change (see Table 3-1). While AREDS supplementation is appropriate for higher grades of dry AMD, there is no strong evidence to recommend such treatment for any of these conditions.[1] Therefore, we offer that patients stop AREDS supplementation, maintain a healthy, well-balanced diet, refrain from smoking, and refrain from vitamin A supplementation in the case of *ABCA4*-retinopathy. We suggest regular use of an Amsler grid, as

CNV is a known complication of many of these conditions. We treat CNV with off-label intra-vitreal anti-VEGF injections using either an as-needed or treat-and-extend algorithm. Finally, we discuss the options for genetic testing when indicated.

Given the prevalence of AMD in the population, its diagnosis will often be correct. However, the recognition of atypical features and appropriate use of questioning and multimodal imaging may reveal an alternate diagnosis that may not only avoid unnecessary treatment, but may also have systemic and/or genetic implications.

References

1. Age-Related Eye Disease Study Research Group. A randomized, placebo-controlled, clinical trial of high dose supplementation with vitamins C and E, beta carotene, and zinc for age-related macular degeneration and vision loss: AREDS report no. 8. *Arch Ophthalmol.* 2001;119(10):1417-1436.
2. Khan KN, Mahroo OA, Khan RS, et al. Differentiating drusen: drusen and drusen-like appearances associated with ageing, age-related macular degeneration, inherited eye disease and other pathological processes. *Prog Retin Eye Res.* 2016;53:70-106.
3. Ferris FL III, Wilkinson CP, Bird A, et al. Clinical classification of age-related macular degeneration. *Ophthalmology.* 2013;120(4):844-851.
4. McBain VA, Egan CA, Pieris SJ, et al. Functional observations in vitamin A deficiency: diagnosis and time course of recovery. *Eye (Lond).* 2007;21(3):367-376.
5. Saksens NT, Fleckenstein M, Schmitz-Valckenberg S, et al. Macular dystrophies mimicking age-related macular degeneration. *Prog Retin Eye Res.* 2014;39:23-57.
6. Gass, JDM. *Stereoscopic Atlas of Macular Diseases: Diagnosis and Treatment,* 4th ed. St. Louis, MO: Mosby; 1997.
7. Westeneng-van Haaften SC, Boon CJ, Cremers FP, et al. Clinical and genetic characteristics of late-onset Stargardt's disease. *Ophthalmology.* 2012;119(6):1199-1210.
8. Fujinami K, Lois N, Davidson AE, et al. A longitudinal study of stargardt disease: clinical and electrophysiologic assessment, progression, and genotype correlations. *Am J Ophthalmol.* 2013;155(6):1075-1088.
9. Radu RA, Yuan Q, Hu J, et al. Accelerated accumulation of lipofuscin pigments in the RPE of a mouse model for ABCA4-mediated retinal dystrophies following Vitamin A supplementation. *Invest Ophthalmol Vis Sci.* 2008;49(9):3821-3829.
10. Francis PJ, Schultz DW, Gregory AM, et al. Genetic and phenotypic heterogeneity in pattern dystrophy. *Br J Ophthalmol.* 2005;89(9):1115-1119.
11. Chan CK, Gass JD, Lin SG. Acute exudative polymorphous vitelliform maculopathy syndrome. *Retina.* 2003;23(4):453-462.
12. Aronow ME, Adamus G, Abu-Asab M, et al. Paraneoplastic vitelliform retinopathy: clinicopathologic correlation and review of the literature. *Surv Ophthalmol.* 2012;57(6):558-564.
13. Nicholson B, Noble J, Forooghian F, Meyerle C. Central serous chorioretinopathy: update on pathophysiology and treatment. *Surv Ophthalmol.* 2013;58(2):103-126.
14. Warrow DJ, Hoang QV, Freund KB. Pachychoroid pigment epitheliopathy. *Retina.* 2013; 33(8):1659-1672.

How Long Are We Going to Have to Keep Doing Frequent Intravitreal Injections—Any Other Options Anytime Soon? What Are We Waiting For?

Margaret A. Greven, MD
Diana V. Do, MD

Intravitreal injections of anti-vascular endothelial growth factor (anti-VEGF) medications are the current standard of care for the treatment of neovascular age-related macular degeneration (AMD), diabetic macular edema (DME), and retinal vein occlusion with macular edema. The 3 currently available drugs in this class are ranibizumab and aflibercept, which are US Food and Drug Administration–approved for the treatment of these conditions, and bevacizumab, which is frequently used off-label. Studies have demonstrated the half-life of these drugs are 7 days for ranibizumab and 9 days for both bevacizumab and aflibercept.[1-3] Ranibizumab and bevacizumab are thought to have a duration of action of approximately 1 month, while aflibercept has been approved for every 1- or 2-month administration.

The goal of treating with these medications is to preserve and improve vision by halting disease activity. The activity of disease is usually determined by the presence of intra- or subretinal fluid, and retinal pigment epithelial detachment associated with choroidal neovascularization in neovascular AMD on optical coherence tomography (OCT) imaging. The 3 common treatment regimens are monthly injections; treat and extend, wherein the interval between injections is gradually increased if the condition remains inactive and shortened to the previous duration at which the patient was inactive, if activity recurs; and as needed, or pro re nata (PRN) injections.

Fekrat S, ed. *Curbside Consultation in Retina: 49 Clinical Questions, Second Edition.* (pp 19-22).
© 2019 SLACK Incorporated

Frequency of Intravitreal Injections

The necessary frequency and duration of intravitreal injections depends on which condition is being treated. In AMD, evidence shows us that there is a continued need for frequent intravitreal injections. The 2-year results of the Comparison of AMD Treatment Trial (CATT), comparing ranibizumab to bevacizumab and monthly injections to PRN injections in neovascular AMD, showed that visual acuity improved over the first 6 months of treatment with monthly or PRN treatment. Improvements were maintained in patients who were continued on a monthly treatment schedule but declined slightly with PRN treatment between year 1 and 2, suggesting more frequent treatment is associated with better visual acuity outcomes.[4] The 5-year results of the CATT follow-up study, an open label follow-up of patients who had been enrolled in the CATT study and received treatment with ranibizumab or bevacizumab at the treating doctor's discretion for an additional 3 years after the first 2 years of the study, showed similar results. Patients received a mean of 4 to 5 injections per year after the first 2 years. However, the mean visual acuity declined an average of 11 letters from year 2 to year 5.[5] It is unclear why these patients lost vision over time as the etiology may be multifactorial. This worsening of vision with reduced treatment frequency could suggest that undertreatment leads to worse vision outcomes and highlights the suggestion that patients continue to require injections even at 5 years after the initiation of treatment. In addition, the development of macular atrophy over time in some of these eyes can also lead to vision loss.

The need for continued frequent injections in neovascular AMD was also supported by the 7-year results of the ANCHOR (Anti-VEGF Antibody for the Treatment of Predominantly Classic Choroidal Neovascularization in AMD), MARINA (Minimally Classic/Occult Trial of the Anti-VEGF Antibody Ranibizumab in the Treatment of Neovascular AMD), and HORIZON (An Open-Label Extension Trial of Ranibizumab for Choroidal Neovascularization Secondary to AMD) studies, which showed that patients who continued to receive the most injections (> 11 injections over a 3-year period) had better visual acuity outcomes.[6] Based on this evidence, in our neovascular AMD patients, we treat aggressively if there is evidence of disease activity on OCT. If all disease activity has resolved, we transition to a treat-and-extend protocol. Once the required interval between injections is established, we continue to treat indefinitely at this interval to prevent recurrent choroidal neovascularization.

The need for continued frequent treatment in neovascular AMD contrasts to the treatment requirement in DME. The 5-year results of the DRCRnet (Diabetic Retinopathy Clinical Research Network) Protocol I showed that patients with DME who received frequent ranibizumab injections, with prompt or deferred laser, during the first year required significantly less injections in subsequent years. These eyes were able to maintain visual acuity improvement despite requiring fewer injections in years 3 through 5.[7] Patients received a mean of 8 or 9 injections in the first year, 2 or 3 injections in the second year, 1 or 2 injections in the third year, and 0 or 1 injection in the fourth year, depending on whether the patient received ranibizumab with prompt or deferred laser. Similarly, the 2-year results of Diabetic Retinopathy Clinical Research Network Protocol T, where patients were randomized to treatment with aflibercept, ranibizumab, or bevacizumab, demonstrated that in the first year patients required an average of 10, 10, or 9 injections respectively, but in the second year, the requirement decreased to 5, 6, or 6, while maintaining sustained visual acuity improvement.[8] Our protocol for treating DME is to treat aggressively initially with monthly injections until the edema resolves and then convert to a PRN treatment approach.

The treatment requirement for retinal vein occlusion with macular edema can vary. The RETAIN study examined outcomes of patients treated for macular edema secondary to branch retinal vein occlusion (BRVO) and central retinal vein occlusion (CRVO) with ranibizumab with a mean follow-up of just over 4 years. Patients with BRVO required an average of about 7 injections the first year, 2.6 injections for the second year, and an average of about 2 injections during both the third and fourth years. About half of BRVO patients still required infrequent injections after 4 years. Patients with CRVO required about 7 injections the first year, 4 injections the second year, 4 injections the third year, and about 3 injections the fourth year. In patients with CRVO, 54% of patients still required frequent injections after 4 years.[9] In our retinal vein occlusion patients, we initially begin with monthly injections until the macular edema has resolved on OCT imaging. Subsequently, we convert to a treat-and-extend protocol to prevent recurrent macular edema or treat on a PRN basis.

Intravitreal steroids are an option to decrease the number of anti-VEGF injections for some eyes with DME and retinal vein occlusion with cystoid macular edema; however, intravitreal steroids may lead to steroid-induced glaucoma and cataract progression in some eyes. Steroid options include preservative-free Triesence (triamcinolone acetonide), Ozurdex (dexamethasone), and Iluvien (fluocinolone acetonide).

Challenges

The evidence tells us that neovascular AMD is a chronic condition that likely requires careful monitoring and frequent treatment. For DME, scientific studies suggest the treatment burden decreases significantly over time. In retinal vein occlusion, eyes with macular edema can require chronic treatment and careful monitoring is necessary. This need for frequent evaluation and possible treatment for these conditions places an enormous burden on our patients. With an aging population and rising prevalence of diabetes, it also places a strain on the health care system. The development of extended-release anti-VEGF treatments holds promise to address these issues in the future.

Future Directions

Several approaches to long-term or extended-release anti-VEGF agents are currently in development. One such approach is implantable reservoir technology that involves surgically attaching a refillable drug reservoir to the sclera to deliver a sustained dose of drug over time. Another approach is encapsulated cell technology which could allow the continuous production of anti-VEGF by immortalized cells within a capsule injected into the vitreous cavity. Still another possible future treatment is gene therapy which could be used to allow the eye to produce its own anti-VEGF. Finally, long-acting anti-VEGF molecules could allow an intravitreal injection to maintain effect for longer than the current duration. Although these approaches to an extended anti-VEGF effect are still under investigation, we believe that within the next 10 years, we will have long-acting anti-VEGF treatments available for our patients. Until then, we will continue with frequent intravitreal injections to give our patients the best visual acuity outcomes.

References

1. Krohne TU, Eter N, Holz FG, Meyer CH. Intraocular pharmacokinetics of bevacizumab after a single intravitreal injection in humans. *Am J Ophthalmol.* 2008;146(4):508-512.
2. Krohne TU, Liu Z, Holz FG, Meyer CH. Intraocular pharmacokinetics of ranibizumab following a single intravitreal injection in humans. *Am J Ophthalmol.* 2012; 154(4):682-686.
3. Do DV. Update on aflibercept pharmacokinetics and treatment of diabetic macular edema. Presented at: Angiogenesis, Exudation, and Degeneration; February 11, 2017. Miami, FL.
4. Martin DF, Maguire MG, Fine SL, et al. Ranibizumab and bevacizumab for treatment of neovascular age-related macular degeneration: two-year results. *Ophthalmology.* 2012;119(7):1388-1398.

5. Maguire MG, Martin DF, Ying GS, et al. Five-year outcomes with anti-vascular endothelial growth factor treatment of neovascular age-related macular degeneration: the comparison of age-related macular degeneration treatments trials. *Ophthalmology.* 2016;123(8):1751-1761.

6. Rofagha S, Bhisitkul RB, Boyer DS, et al. Seven-year outcomes in ranibizumab-treated patients in ANCHOR, MARINA, and HORIZON: a multicenter cohort study (SEVEN-UP). *Ophthalmology.* 2013;120(11):2292-2299.

7. Elman MJ, Ayalla A, Bressler NM, et al. Intravitreal ranibizumab for diabetic macular edema with prompt versus deferred laser treatment: 5-year randomized trial results. *Ophthalmology.* 2015;122(2):375-381.

8. Wells, JA, Glassman AR, Ayala AR, et al. Aflibercept, bevacizumab, or ranibizumab for diabetic macular edema: two-year results from a comparative effectiveness randomized clinical trial. *Ophthalmology.* 2016;123(6):1351-1359.

9. Campochiaro PA, Sophie R, Pearlman J, et al. Longterm outcomes in patients with retinal vein occlusion treated with ranibizumab: the RETAIN study. *Ophthalmology.* 2014;121(1):209-219.

ANYTHING COMING DOWN THE PIKE YET FOR DRY AGE-RELATED MACULAR DEGENERATION?

Jose Mauricio Botto Garcia, MD, MSc

Philip J. Rosenfeld, MD, PhD

Age-related macular degeneration (AMD) is a leading cause of severe irreversible vision loss among the elderly worldwide.[1-4] Severe vision loss is a feature of late AMD, which includes geographic atrophy (GA) and exudative AMD.[1] The only approved, effective, injectable therapies solely target the exudative form of AMD, which comprises about 20% of late AMD.[1] Exudative AMD is treated by injecting inhibitors of vascular endothelial growth factor into the eye, but even in the best of circumstances, the injections dry the exudative AMD, which may continue to slowly advance with significant vision loss over time.[5] Currently, there are no effective therapies that are approved for the treatment of late, dry AMD (ie, GA) and there are no effective therapies that can slow the progression of intermediate dry AMD, which is characterized by drusen and pigmentary abnormalities.[1-3,6,7]

GA is characterized by the localized loss of macular photoreceptors, retinal pigment epithelium (RPE), and choriocapillaris.[2,6,8-11] While the focus of GA has been shown to arise from drusen[12] and then enlarge over time, it is also possible for GA to develop in the absence of drusen.[4] While the genetics of AMD suggest a role for the abnormal regulation of the complement pathway as an underlying cause of the disease,[2,6] the exact mechanism by which complement causes AMD remains elusive.[6] The most significant association exists between at-risk complement alleles and the presence and growth of drusen;[3] however, large epidemiological studies have not yet found an association between at-risk complement alleles and the increased growth of GA.[11] Despite the lack of a compelling association between complement at-risk alleles and the growth of GA, numerous studies have used complement inhibitors in an attempt to slow the enlargement of GA. In addition, other strategies have been studied in an attempt to slow the enlargement of GA,[2,6,13] and these strategies include visual cycle modulation, beta-amyloid inhibition, protection against oxidative damage, and neuroprotection.[2,7,14]

Fekrat S, ed. *Curbside Consultation in Retina: 49 Clinical Questions, Second Edition.* (pp 23-30).
© 2019 SLACK Incorporated

The most frequently used clinical trial endpoint for the study of nonexudative AMD is to study a drug's ability to slow the enlargement of GA over time.[3] While other endpoints have been proposed that involve slowing the enlargement of drusen in intermediate AMD and slowing the progression of intermediate AMD to late AMD, only one drug study to date has investigated one of these alternative endpoints.[3] While the limited scope of this review precludes a detailed description of all studied therapies to date, the drugs that follow are either currently in clinical trials or will soon enter trials for the treatment of dry AMD.

Complement Pathway Inhibition

As local inflammation and complement activation are implicated as a cause of AMD, inhibition of the complement pathway has been studied as a therapeutic approach.[6,9,14,15] Genentech/Roche investigated lampalizumab, a monoclonal antibody fragment (Fab) against complement factor D that prevents the activation and amplification of the alternative complement pathway.[15] The Phase II MAHALO (A Study to Evaluate the Long-Term Safety and Tolerability of Lampalizumab (FCFD4514S) in Patients With Geographic Atrophy Who Have Completed Genentech-Sponsored Lampalizumab Studies) study demonstrated a 20% reduction in the rate of GA progression after 18 months with monthly lampalizumab intravitreal injections (10 mg) compared to sham injections.[3,6,16] While this result did not show conventional statistical significance, they did show a statistically significant reduction of 44% in a subgroup analysis of patients carrying an at-risk allele in the complement factor I locus. Given that this significant finding was found in a small subgroup, confirmation of this association between complement factor I, reduction in GA progression, and lampalizumab inhibition is needed.[16] Two parallel, multicenter, international Phase III studies with lampalizumab, known as *CHROMA* (A Study to Assess the Efficacy and Safety of Lampalizumab Administered Intravitreally to Patients With Geographic Atrophy Secondary to AMD) and *SPECTRI* (A Study Investigating the Safety and Efficacy of Lampalizumab Intravitreal Injections in Participants With Geographic Atrophy Secondary to AMD), were performed. To be enrolled in these studies, patients had to have bilateral GA containing a banded pattern of hyperautofluorescence. These patients were then randomized to receive lampalizumab (10 mg) injections every 4 or 6 weeks or a sham injection. Unfortunately, Genentech/Roche announced that both SPECTRI and CHROMA failed to reach the primary endpoint and the studies were stopped.[15]

Another complement inhibitor in clinical trials, which is known as *LFG316* (Novartis), is an antibody against the complement component 5 (C5) of the complement pathway. C5 inhibition should effectively inhibit late stage complement activation and prevent membrane attach complex (MAC) formation. In a Phase IIb study, intravitreal LFG316 did not slow the enlargement of GA when compared with a sham injection. Then, LFG316 was combined with CLG561, a drug that inhibits another complement pathway protein known as *properdin*. Although no official report has been released, this combination therapy study apparently failed to meet its endpoint. Zimura (avacincaptad pegol) is another inhibitor of C5, but this drug is a chemically synthesized aptamer. Zimura is being evaluated currently in a Phase II/III study.[7] APL-2 (Apellis Pharmaceuticals) is a pegylated peptide inhibitor of complement factor C3, which effectively inhibits both the classical and alternative pathways of complement activation. In the prospective, randomized, multicenter, sham-controlled, single-masked Phase II clinical trial, subjects were randomized to receive intravitreal APL-2 (15 mg) vs sham-injection every month or every other month over 12 months with final follow-up at 18 months. Apellis recently announced that APL-2 met its primary endpoint at 12 months.[17] Monthly intravitreal injections of APL-2 showed a 29% ($P=0.008$) reduction in the rate of GA lesion growth compared with sham. In the group treated every other month, a 20% ($P=0.067$) reduction was observed. In addition, a post hoc analysis showed that APL-2's effect was greater in the second 6 months of the study compared with the first 6 months, with a reduction in growth rate of 47% ($P < 0.001$) with monthly administration, and a reduction of 33% ($P = 0.01$) with every other month administration. Follow-up continued for 18 months and after 18 months, the growth rate of GA increased off therapy and returned to the rate observed with the sham treated group.[18] A gene therapy strategy for the inhibition of complement activation is being investigated in a Phase I clinical trial that is using an adeno-associated virus that expresses a naturally occurring cell surface inhibitor of MAC known as *CD59*. This study, which is investigating a single intravitreal injection of HMR59 (Hemera BioSciences Inc.), is currently enrolling patients.[19] The antibiotic doxycycline is also under study. This drug has demonstrated anti-inflammatory properties and has also been shown to prevent complement activation. This study, which is investigating 40 mg oral daily Oracea (doxycycline) for 24 months, is currently enrolling patients (Table 5-1).[20]

Neuroprotection

Brimonidine tartrate is a drug approved by the US Food and Drug Administration for the treatment of glaucoma and it has also been shown to have neuroprotection properties.[7,14] Following a small Phase II study that showed encouraging results with brimonidine tartrate delivered through an intravitreal implant, a larger Phase II clinical trial was started. In this trial, patients will be treated with a 400 μg brimonidine implant, injected every 3 months for 24 months, and compared to a sham group.[14] Unfortunately, the study has been stopped, but the results have not been released (Table 5-2).

Mitochondrial Bioenergetics

Elamipretide (Stealth BioTherapeutics) is a compound designed to selectively target cardiolipin involved with the electron transport chain and oxidative phosphorylation of mitochondria in an attempt to improve cellular bioenergetics. The ReCLAIM (An Open-Label, Phase 1 Clinical Study to Evaluate the Safety and Tolerability of Subcutaneous Elamipretide in Subjects With Intermediate Age-Related Macular Degeneration) Phase I study is evaluating elamipretide for intermediate AMD and late AMD with nonsubfoveal GA. Eligible subjects will receive 40 mg of elamipretide administered as a once daily 1.0 mL subcutaneous injection for 12 weeks. Patients with any evidence of central GA will be excluded.[21] This study is currently enrolling patients (Table 5-3).

Stem Cell Therapy

Another promising strategy in the treatment of GA is stem cell therapy.[7] Stem cell transplantation could lead to prevention of disease progression, either by replacing damaged cells or providing trophic factors to prevent degeneration. Another less likely possibility is that stem cells could cause regeneration of RPE and photoreceptors that have been damaged. Currently, differentiated human embryonic stem cells (hESC) and the induced pluripotent stem cells are being investigated for the treatment of late-stage AMD.

In 2012, Schwartz and colleagues published the first description of hESC transplantation into human subjects with retinal disease.[22] These cells had been fully differentiated into RPE prior to their transplantation into the subretinal space adjacent to the area of GA.[10,21,23]

Table 5-1
Modulation of Inflammation

Drug	Mechanism of Action	Delivery	Clinical Trial Identifier	Phase	Company Name	Status
FCFD4514S (Lampalizumab)	Anti-factor D Fab	Intravitreal injection	NCT02247479 NCT02247531	III	Genentech	Failed
Zimura	Aptamer; inhibits complement factor C5	Intravitreal injection	NCT02686658	II/III	Ophthotech	Ongoing
CLG561 + LFG316	Human antibody against Properdin ± antibody against C5	Intravitreal injection	NCT02515942	IIb	Novartis	Failed
APL-2	Pegylated cyclic peptide against C3	Intravitreal injection	NCT02503332	II	Apellis Pharmaceuticals	Positive
APL-2	Pegylated cyclic peptide against C3	Intravitreal injection	NCT03525600 NCT03525613	III	Apellis Pharmaceuticals	Not yet recruiting
Oracea (tetracycline derivative-doxycycline)	Suppresses inflammation	Oral	NCT01782989	II/III	University of Virginia	Enrolling
HMR59 (gene therapy)	Inhibits MAC	Single intravitreal injection	NCT03144999	I	Hemera BioSciences	Active; not recruiting

Table 5-2

Neuroprotection

Drug	Mechanism of Action	Delivery	Clinical Trial Identifier	Phase	Company Name	Status
Brimonidine tartrate	α-2 adrenergic receptor agonist	Intravitreal implant	NCT02087085	II	Allergan	Failed

Table 5-3

Modulation of Mitochondrial Bioenergetics

Drug	Mechanism of Action	Delivery	Clinical Trial Identifier	Phase	Company Name	Status
Elamipretide	Inhibits mitichondrial dysfunction in the RPE	Subcutaneous	NCT02848313	I	Stealth	Completed; Phase II being planned

Safety and tolerability of these subretinally transplanted hESC-derived RPE were confirmed in this Phase I study, which enrolled 9 patients with dry AMD who were followed up for approximately 22 months. The results of this study showed medium- to long-term safety, graft survival, and the possibility of biological activity based on improved visual acuity. This study demonstrated that hESC-derived cells could provide a potentially safe new source of cells for the treatment of various unmet medical disorders requiring tissue repair or replacement. A Phase II study is currently being organized. Cell Cure Neurosciences Ltd. is performing a similar trial using hESCs differentiated into RPE.

The feasibility and safety of delivering hESC-derived RPE on a parylene membrane (CPCB-RPE1) is being studied in an ongoing Phase I/II program. hESC-RPE on parylene membranes have demonstrated improved survival with an intact RPE monolayer graft by simulating the support of a Bruch membrane compared with cell suspensions.[24] This study is currently enrolling patients (Table 5-4).

Summary

Currently, there are no treatments to slow the appearance and progression of GA, which is a major cause of irreversible blindness from nonexudative AMD worldwide. However, numerous drugs and several cell therapy strategies are being investigated. Within the next few years, we may have treatments that will at least slow the relentless enlargement of GA and slow the vision loss associated with late nonexudative AMD.

Table 5-4

Stem Cells Therapy

Drug	Mechanism of Action	Delivery	Clinical Trial Identifier	Phase	Company Name	Status
hESC–RPE	hESC–derived RPE	Subretinal injection	Pending	Ib/II	Astellas	Unknown
CPCB-RPE1	hESC–derived RPE (parylene membrane)	Subretinal implantation	NCT02590692	I/II	Regenerative Patch Technologies	Active; not recruiting
hESC–RPE	hESC–derived RPE	Intraocular injection	NCT02286089	I/II	Cell Cure Neurosciences	Recruiting

References

1. Ferris FL III, Wilkinson CP, Bird A, et al. Clinical classification of age-related macular degeneration. *Ophthalmology*. 2013;120(4):844-851.
2. Holz FG, Strauss EC, Schmitz-Valckenberg S, van Lookeren Campagne M. Geographic atrophy: clinical features and potential therapeutic approaches. *Ophthalmology*. 2014;121(5):1079-1091.
3. Schaal KB, Rosenfeld PJ, Gregori G, et al. Anatomic clinical trial endpoints for nonexudative age-related macular degeneration. *Ophthalmology*. 2016;123(5):1060-1079.
4. Spaide RF. Age-related choroidal atrophy. *Am J Ophthalmol*. 2009;147(5):801-810.
5. Grunwald JE, Pistilli M, Daniel E, et al. Incidence and growth of geographic atrophy during 5 years of comparison of age-related macular degeneration treatments trials. *Ophthalmology*. 2017;124(1):97-104.
6. Boyer DS, Schmidt-Erfurth U, van Lookeren Campagne M, et al. The pathophysiology of geographic atrophy secondary to age-related macular degeneration and the complement pathway as a therapeutic target. *Retina*. 2017;37(5):819-835. doi: 10.1097/IAE.0000000000001392.
7. Sacconi R, Corbelli E, Querques L, et al. A review of current and future management of geographic atrophy. *Ophthalmol Ther*. 2017;6(1):69–77.
8. Klein R, Lee KE, Gangnon RE, Klein BE. Incidence of visual impairment over a 20-year period: the Beaver Dam Eye Study. *Ophthalmology*. 2013;120(6):1210-1219.
9. Zarbin MA. Current concepts in the pathogenesis of age-related macular degeneration. *Arch Ophthalmol*. 2004;122(4):598-614.
10. Schwartz SD, Regillo CD, Lam BL, et al. Human embryonic stem cell-derived retinal pigment epithelium in patients with age-related macular degeneration and Stargardt's macular dystrophy: follow-up of two open-label phase 1/2 studies. *Lancet*. 2017;385(9967):509-516.
11. Grassmann F, Fleckenstein M, Chew EY, et al. Clinical and genetic factors associated with progression of geographic atrophy lesions in age-related macular degeneration. *PLoS One*. 2015;10(5):e0126636.
12. Wu Z, Luu CD, Ayton LN, et al. Optical coherence tomography-defined changes preceding the development of drusen-associated atrophy in age-related macular degeneration. *Ophthalmology*. 2014;121(12):2415-2422.
13. Ambati J, Atkinson JP, Gelfand BD. Immunology of age-related macular degeneration. *Nat Rev Immunol*. 2013;13(6):438-451.
14. Patel HR, Eichenbaum D. Geographic atrophy: clinical impact and emerging treatments. *Ophthalmic Surg Lasers Imaging Retina*. 2015;46(1):8-13
15. Holz FG, Busbee B, Chew EY, et al. Efficacy and safety of Lampalizumab for geographic atrophy due to age-related macular degeneration CHROMA and SPECTRI phase 3 randomized clinical trials. *JAMA Ophthalmol*. 2018. [Epub ahead of print]. doi: 10.1001/jamaophthalmol.2018.1544
16. Yaspan BL, Williams DF, Holz FG, et al. Targeting factor D of the alternative complement pathway reduces geographic atrophy progression secondary to age-related macular degeneration. *Science Transl Med*. 2017;9(395): pii: eaaf1443.
17. Apellis Pharmaceuticals. Apellis Pharmaceuticals announces that APL-2 Met its Primary Endpoint in a phase 2 study in patients with geographic atrophy, an advanced form of age-related macular degeneration. www.apellis.com/pdfs/Press%20Release%20FILLY%2012%20Month%20Results%20FINAL%20FINAL%20170823.pdf. Published August 24, 2017. Accessed June 11, 2018.
18. Apellis Pharmaceuticals. Apellis Pharmaceuticals announces 18-month results of phase 2 study (FILLY) of APL-2 in geographic atrophy. http://investors.apellis.com/news-releases/news-release-details/apellis-pharmaceuticals-announces-18-month-results-phase-2-study. Published February 22, 2018. Accessed June 11, 2018.
19. Hemera Biosciences. www.hemerabiosciences.com. Published 2018. Accessed June 7, 2018.
20. Clinical Study to Evaluate Treatment with Oracea for Geographic Atrophy (TOGA). *ClinicalTrials*. https://clinicaltrials.gov/ct2/show/NCT01782989. Updated August 24, 2017. Accessed June 4, 2018.
21. An OpenLabel, Phase 1 Clinical Study to Evaluate the Safety and Tolerability of Subcutaneous Elamipretide in Subjects With Intermediate AgeRelated Macular Degeneration. *ClinicalTrials*. https://clinicaltrials.gov/ct2/show/NCT02848313?term=Stealth&rank=23. 2017. Updated September 6, 2017. Accessed June 8, 2018.
22. Schwartz SD, Hubschman JP, Heilwell G, et al. Embryonic stem cell trials for macular degeneration: a preliminary report. *Lancet*. 2012;379(9817):713-720.
23. Schwartz SD, Tan G, Hosseini H, Nagiel A. Subretinal transplantation of embryonic stem cell-derived retinal pigment epithelium for the treatment of macular degeneration: an assessment at 4 years. *Invest Ophthalmol Vis Sci*. 2016;57(5):1-9.
24. Diniz B, Thomas P, Thomas B, et al. Subretinal implantation of retinal pigment epithelial cells derived from human embryonic stem cells: improved survival when implanted as a monolayer. *Invest Ophthalmol Vis Sci*. 2013;54(7):5087-5096.

ARE WE EVER GOING TO USE STEM CELLS? FOR WHAT? WHAT'S THE SCOOP?

Steven D. Schwartz, MD

Progress in the diagnosis and treatment of retinal disease is advancing at an unprecedented pace, yet there remains a significant societal burden of untreatable blindness resulting from disorders of the retina. This includes relatively common diseases, such as dry age-related macular degeneration, and less common conditions, such as retinitis pigmentosa and Stargardt disease. Stem cell-based strategies represent a promising therapeutic modality and catalyst for research. Stem cell-derived retinal pigment epithelium has already been transplanted into humans with central macular atrophy, and human photoreceptor transplantation is likely on the horizon. In addition, a variety of stem cell derivatives have shown promise as neuroprotective agents when transplanted into the eye.

Gene and cell therapy have the potential to prevent, halt, or reverse diseases of the retina in patients with currently incurable blinding diseases. Over the past 2 decades, major advances in our understanding of the pathobiologic basis of retinal diseases, coupled with growth of gene transfer and cell transplantation biotechnologies, have created optimism that previously blinding retinal conditions may be treatable. However, while gene therapies may be nearing approval, stem cell or regenerative cell therapies are likely at least 5 to 7 years away from regulatory approval at the time of this chapter.

In today's world, however, patients are exposed to media and internet reports that are, at best, lacking nuance and detail and, at worst, intentionally deceptive. Unavoidably, every ophthalmologist has been or will be asked about stem cell therapies repeatedly. One of our roles as physicians and surgeons is to protect our patients from charlatans and scams that jeopardize safety for profit. My answer to each patient remains, "Stem cells are not approved and may be dangerous. You are not a candidate despite what you may hear or read online. Any use of unapproved therapies will likely preclude future treatment with well-studied therapies. If they ask you to pay, walk away."

Fekrat S, ed. *Curbside Consultation in Retina: 49 Clinical Questions, Second Edition.* (pp 31-34).
© 2019 SLACK Incorporated

When health care providers ask, "What's the scoop? Will we ever legitimately use stem cells for eye disease?" the appropriate response is, "Probably, but I'm an optimist." A number of critical points deserve emphasis:

- There are currently no US Food and Drug Administration (FDA)–approved stem cell therapies.

- Risks of stem cell transplantation include, but are not limited to, loss of life, loss of eye, loss of vision, and severe systemic immune disease, among others.

- Despite the lack of proven, approved therapies, unproven, for-profit "stem cell therapies" are being sold to patients, jeopardizing both patient safety and scientific credibility.

Our mission as physicians and surgeons is to prevent and reduce human suffering and to protect patient safety. Impending blindness is certainly a source of suffering, and as such, creates a sense of urgency when the underlying condition is untreatable. This urgency coupled with the promise of stem cell biology and media interest in ongoing, legitimate clinical trials has led to a perfect storm wherein any number of problematic, dangerous, for-profit programs are leveraging desperation, poor public understanding, imprecise media coverage, and little or no regulatory involvement. In a perfect world, all clinical trials would be constructed with patient safety and respect for the scientific method as the guiding priority, and treatments would be guided by reliable data and high-level evidence. Unfortunately, the public's insatiable desire for anything stem cell and irrational beliefs that stem cells cure everything have created a market for untested, unproven, unregulated, and often baseless "therapies." "Often, these cells…are being used in practice on the basis of minimal clinical evidence of safety or efficacy, sometimes with the claim that they constitute revolutionary treatments for various conditions."[1] To illustrate the magnitude of this issue, in 2015, there were 570 clinics marketing stem cell treatment directly to consumers. Documented cases of harm, including iatrogenic blindness and pain necessitating bilateral enucleation, have prompted the American Academy of Ophthalmology (AAO) to ask, "How does the physician community distinguish legitimate clinical investigation from uncontrolled commercial use in the guise of investigation?"

Public misperceptions include:

- "Stem cells can cure anything."

- "Stem cell therapy is no/low risk."

- "If an institutional review board has approved it, it's safe and probably going to be effective."

- "If not FDA-regulated, it is FDA-approved."

- "If it is listed on clinicaltrials.gov, it has been reviewed and approved by the National Institutes of Health."

To help clarify or distinguish real science from the rest, the International Society for Stem Cell Research has pointed out the following warning signs:

- Same stem cells for multiple diseases

- Source of stem cells unclear

- No formal treatment protocol

- Claims based on patient testimonials

- Claims of no risk

Most importantly, I tell patients, "If you have to pay (to 'participate in research'), stay away." In fact, both the AAO and the International Society for Stem Cell Research agree that if the treatment costs money, it is likely illegitimate and may jeopardize patient safety in an irreversible manner. The AAO position as of 2018 is positive, "The potential of stem-cell based technologies hold promise for the repair, restoration and regeneration of dysfunctional cells in the eye, yet significant challenges remain. These treatments appear to offer hope to patients who may have limited options for recovery of vision, including patients with age-related macular degeneration, retinitis pigmentosa and Stargardt disease."[2] "The Academy believes that, in the interests of public health and patient safety, the FDA should continue to investigate unlicensed clinics that offer unapproved stem-cell therapy and to take appropriate regulatory actions. These treatments require further scientific evaluation to assure their safety and effectiveness to the public in well-conducted clinical trials under the aegis of the FDA."[2] As a translational researcher committed to the scientific method, patient safety, and innovation, I wholeheartedly support the AAO's efforts to support the science, promote rigorous scientific method with societal impact, and protect patients as its priority. The context or framework in which not only science is conducted, but the environment in which it is interpreted and translated into clinical practice is, and should be, the purview of organized ophthalmology.

Summary

Stem cell-based therapies hold promise and may open pathways towards reduced suffering from visual loss. Unfortunately, progress toward these goals may be impeded by poorly designed, for-profit, dangerous "therapies" that are not based on rigorous science. Optimistically, with good teamwork, collaboration, and commitment to the scientific method, the legitimate use of stem cells in ophthalmology may be just around the corner.

Acknowledgment

Special recognition to Dr. David Parke and his team at the American Academy of Ophthalmology for their support and leadership.

References

1. Anson P. Stem cell therapy: hope or hype for pain patients? Pain News Network. https://www.painnewsnetwork.org/stories/2016/12/1/stem-cell-therapy-hope-or-hype-for-pain-patients. Published December 1, 2016. Accessed July 17, 2018.
2. AAO Quality of Care Secretariat, Hoskins Center for Quality Eye Care. Intraocular stem cell therapy—2016. https://www.aao.org/clinical-statement/intraocular-stem-cell-therapy. Published June 2016. Accessed July 17, 2018.

Suggested Readings

Parke DW II, Lum F, McLeod SD. Stem cell treatment: think twice if they ask for payment. *Ophthalmology*. 2016;123(10S):S62-S63. doi: 10.1016/j.ophtha.2016.07.039.
Marks PW, Witten CM, Califf, RM. Clarifying stem-cell therapy's benefits and risks. *N Engl J Med*. 2017;376(11):1007-1009.
MacLaren RE, Bennett J, Schwartz SD. Gene therapy and stem cell transplantation in retinal disease: the new frontier. *Ophthalmology*. 2016;123(10S):S98-S106. doi: 10.1016/j.ophtha.2016.06.041.
Rakoczy EP, Lai CM, Magno AL, et al. Gene therapy with recombinant adeno-associated vectors for neovascular age-related macular degeneration: 1 year follow-up of a phase 1 randomized clinical trial. *Lancet*. 2015;386(10011):2395-2403.
Schwartz SD, Hubschman JP, Heilweil G, et al. Embryonic stem cell trials for macular degeneration: a preliminary report. *Lancet*. 2012;379(9817):713-720.

Figure 7-1. The set-up of the room is essential to obtaining a good B-scan; the patient should be reclined, the machine should be near the patient's head, and the examiner should be seated.

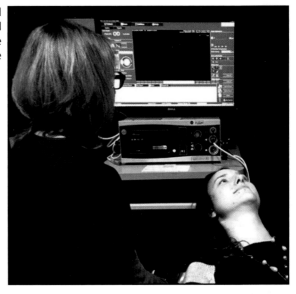

Third, the marker on the probe (white line) represents the upper portion of the echogram (Figure 7-2A) and changing the position of the marker changes the direction of the sound beam as it travels through the eye. The center of the sound beam provides the best detail of ocular structures. When the posterior segment is being evaluated, the probe is placed opposite the area to be examined and the patient should be looking in the direction where the sound beam is aimed. If the patient's eyes are closed, it can be difficult for the patient and the examiner to know where the patient is looking. The eye can be examined in different planes to provide a 3D perspective using 2D images.

- Transverse scans provide cross-sectional views opposite of where the probe is positioned. The sound beam is aligned perpendicular to the globe wall and a thin section (2.0 mm in thickness) of tissue is examined along 6 clock hours (see Figure 7-2). To look at the superior or inferior fundus, the marker should be directed toward the patient's nose. These are known as *horizontal transverse scans*. To look at the nasal or temporal fundus, the marker should be directed toward the 12 o'clock position. These are known as *vertical transverse scans*.

- When performing transverse scans, place the probe on the eye with the marker directed in the correct location and overlap the corneal limbus until you see the shadow of the optic nerve. Then, slowly shift the probe from the limbus into the fornix or toward the canthus, being sure to aim the sound into the periphery. Failing to move the probe limits the areas of the globe being examined. Failure to move the probe in this fashion often results in missed findings in the far periphery.

- The center of the image provides the best detail of intraocular structures. If, during your vertical and horizontal transverse scans, you see something that you want to evaluate better, but it is not in the center of the image, you can adjust the probe face and the marker to obtain an *oblique transverse scan*. For instance, during a horizontal transverse scan toward superior in the right eye, you see something more toward the bottom of the image (Figures 7-3A and 7-3B). Moving the probe face to the 4:30 location with the marker directed toward superonasal directs the center of the sound beam superotemporal and the area you were seeing in the previous scan is now in the center of the screen (Figures 7-3C and 7-3D). Shifting the probe from the limbus to the fornix is essential to evaluate the area from posterior to anteriorly.

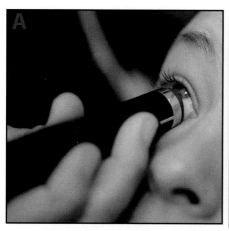
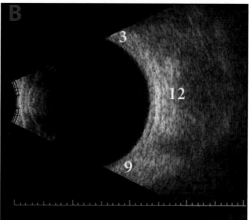

Figure 7-2. (A) Probe position to evaluate the superior fundus; the patient is looking up toward the eyebrows, the probe face is placed on the inferior globe wall, and the marker is directed toward the nose. (B) Horizontal transverse scan toward the superior fundus. The sound beam is moving horizontally (back and forth toward the marker). A thin section of tissue, about 2 mm in diameter, is viewed along 6 clock hours. As the marker is directed toward the nose, nasal, or 3 o'clock, is at the top of the image. Opposite 3 o'clock is 9 o'clock at the bottom of the image, and the center of the sound beam is aimed at 12 o'clock in the center of the image.

- *Longitudinal scans* provide radial views of the intraocular areas opposite of where the probe face is positioned. The sound beam is aligned parallel to the globe wall and a thin section of tissue along a single meridian or clock hour is obtained (Figure 7-4). The probe face is placed opposite the area you want to examine and the marker on the probe should be placed near the corneal limbus, aimed at the clock hour you intend to evaluate. The patient should still be instructed to look in the area opposite the face of the probe. To visualize mobility during longitudinal scans, ask the patient to look straight and then back to the area you are scanning.

- For *axial scans*, instruct the patient to look straight up. In the obtained image, the lens and optic nerve should be in the center of the screen. Vertical scans (Figure 7-5) show the superior (above the nerve shadow) and inferior (below the nerve shadow) posterior pole. Horizontal scans show the nasal (above the nerve) and temporal (below the nerve) posterior pole. *Oblique axial scans* can be performed by directing the marker to one of the superior oblique clock hours.

I generally teach individuals to follow *SNIT* as the scanning sequence: Vertical and horizontal transverse scans to *S*uperior, *N*asal, *I*nferior, and *T*emporal quadrants. Set the gain on the machine to the maximum setting to look for fine vitreous opacities. Adjust the gain setting to improve the resolution when highly reflective pathology is noted. Maximum or high gain shows fine vitreous echoes. Decreasing the gain improves the resolution of the ocular coats (retina, choroid, and sclera).

Place the probe face near the corneal limbus inferiorly with the marker directed toward the nose. The sound beam is now aimed toward the superior fundus. Locate the shadow of the optic nerve and then slowly shift the probe from the limbus (beam aimed posteriorly) to the fornix (beam aimed toward the periphery). If the vitreous cavity is not echo free, instruct the patient to keep looking up, and then look left and right to assess mobility of any echoes.

Next, instruct the patient to look nasally. Place the probe on the temporal globe near the corneal limbus with the marker directed toward the 12 o'clock position. The sound beam is now aimed toward the nasal fundus. Locate the shadow of the optic nerve then shift the probe from the limbus to the fornix. If you want to evaluate mobility, ask the patient to keep looking toward his or her nose, and then look up and down. Next, ask the patient to look down, place the probe

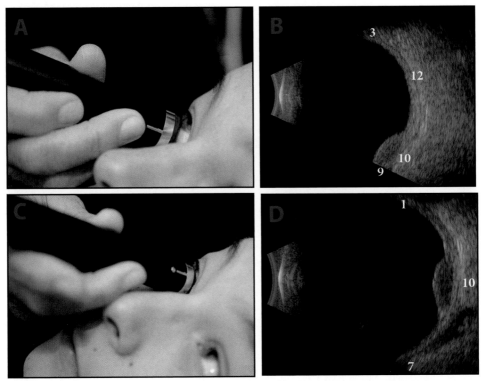

Figure 7-3. (A) At the beginning of the screening process, the patient is looking up toward the eyebrows. The probe face is placed on the inferior globe wall, and the marker is directed toward the nose. (B) The right B-scan image shows a lesion toward the bottom of the image, or superotemporally. As the sound beam is not aimed perpendicular to this area, the examiner will not be able to obtain complete topographic information about the lesion. (C) Adjust the position of the probe face to the inferonasal position with the marker directed toward 1 o'clock; now the center of the sound beam is aimed toward 10 o'clock (superotemporally). (D) The B-scan image now shows the entire borders of the mass-like lesion. The top of the image represents the location of the marker at 1 o'clock, the center of the sound beam is aimed toward 10 o'clock, where the lesion is located and the bottom of the screen shows the 7 o'clock region. Remember that the center of the sound beam provides the best detail.

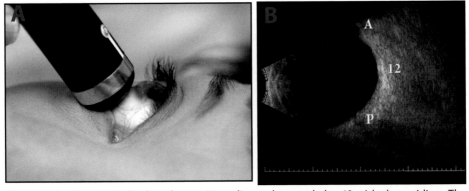

Figure 7-4. (A) Longitudinal probe position directed toward the 12 o'clock meridian. The patient is still looking up, the probe face is placed on the inferior globe wall, and the marker is near the inferior limbus, directed toward 12 o'clock. (B) Longitudinal B-scan image showing the entire 12 o'clock meridian from the periphery (A) to the posterior pole (P). The shadow of the optic nerve should be near the bottom of the image.

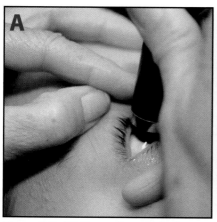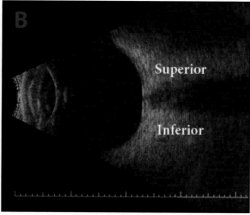

Figure 7-5. (A) The probe positioning to perform a vertical axial scan. The patient should be looking straight up. The probe is placed gently on the cornea with the marker directed toward 12 o'clock. (B) Vertical axial B-scan image. The lens and optic nerve should be centered in the image. The superior posterior pole is the area above the optic nerve shadow. The inferior posterior pole is the area below the optic nerve shadow.

on the superior globe near the corneal limbus, with the marker directed toward the nose. The sound beam is now aimed toward the inferior fundus. Locate the shadow of the optic nerve and then shift the probe from the limbus to the fornix to evaluate the inferior globe from the posterior pole to the periphery. Finally, ask the patient to look temporally. Place the probe on the nasal globe near the corneal limbus with the marker directed toward the 12 o'clock position. The sound beam is now aimed toward the temporal fundus. Locate the shadow of the optic nerve and then shift the probe from the limbus to the fornix. Having the patient move his or her eye in the direction of the sound beam during the screening process may provide additional useful information. Once the entire globe has been evaluated using transverse scans, evaluate the globe using longitudinal scans. You can do this along any single clock hour to evaluate from the posterior pole to the periphery. If the transverse scans show little pathology, I suggest doing longitudinal scans toward nasal and temporal. To do this, ask the patient to look toward nasal. Place the probe on the temporal globe with the marker directed toward the temporal corneal limbus. The sound beam will be aimed toward the nasal clock hour (3 o'clock in the right eye and 9 o'clock in the left eye). In the image, locate the shadow of the optic nerve at the bottom of the screen. If you need to see more of the periphery, pull the probe more toward the fornix, keeping the marker directed toward nasal. Next, have the patient look temporally. Place the probe on the nasal globe with the marker directed toward the nasal limbus. The sound beam will be aimed toward the temporal clock hour (9 o'clock in the right eye and 3 o'clock in the left eye). In the image, the nerve should be at the bottom of the screen.

As a rule, if I intend to describe a finding in my report, I make sure I have an image to support the description. It is important to label your ultrasound scans when you are saving them so that they can be correlated with the exam and accurately repeated for comparison on follow up visits. Scans captured along 3 main axes of the globe—transverse, longitudinal, and axial—should be labelled as follows:

- Transverse scans: Label with the clock hour that is in the center of the screen and an estimated location along that clock hour (ie, 12 P [posterior pole], PE [posterior to equator], E [equator], EA [anterior to equator], O [ora], CB [ciliary body]).

- Longitudinal scans: Label with an L and the clock hour being examined (ie, L12, L1, L2, L3).

- Axial scans: Label VAX (vertical), HAX (horizontal) or, if you are performing an oblique axial, label the image using the clock hour where the marker is directed (ie, 1:30 AX).

There are several instances where patients may be followed with serial ultrasound examinations. Ideally, the same machine and same image settings should be used during repeat examinations to provide the most accurate representation of previous findings and/or changes.

Summary

Following a systematic approach with a prescribed screening sequence will yield the most useful information and assure that all areas of the globe have been examined in an efficient and repeatable manner.

WHEN DO I REFER A PATIENT WITH A BRANCH RETINAL ARTERY OCCLUSION OR CENTRAL RETINAL ARTERY OCCLUSION, WHAT IS THE WORK-UP, AND WHAT ARE THE TREATMENT OPTIONS?

Todd R. Klesert, MD, PhD

Although a thorough systemic work-up may not always yield a causative etiology, there is no such thing as an idiopathic retinal artery occlusion (RAO). RAOs are often the first manifestation of a larger, potentially serious, systemic condition that may require treatment, and therefore always warrant further evaluation. In my opinion, this is best accomplished in conjunction with the patient's primary care physician.

The causes of RAO are many, but may be grouped into a few primary categories: embolic, coagulopathic, inflammatory/autoimmune, traumatic, infectious, and structural. Overall, *embolism* is the most frequent cause of arterial occlusion (Figure 8-1). For patients over the age of 40, atherosclerotic plaques in the aorta, carotid, and ophthalmic arteries are the most frequent source of emboli. In patients under 40, cardiac sources predominate: valvular disease (including septic emboli from endocarditis), arrhythmia, wall motion abnormalities, myxoma, and septal defects, such as a patent foramen ovale in the setting of deep venous thrombosis.

The suspicion for coagulopathy should increase as patient age decreases. Many of the well-established genetic risk factors for venous thrombosis (ie, Factor V Leiden mutation, prothrombin G20210A gene mutation, protein C and S deficiency, activated protein C resistance, antithrombin III deficiency) are less strongly correlated as risk factors for arterial thrombosis.[1] I therefore do not routinely order these expensive laboratory tests unless the more common causes of RAO have been excluded, or the past medical and/or family histories are suggestive of a hereditary thrombophilia. Procoagulant factors that have been associated with arterial thrombosis include antiphospholipid antibodies, anticardiolipin antibodies, elevated homocysteine levels, sickle cell disease, malignancy, blood dyscrasia, pregnancy, and oral contraceptive use (particularly in conjunction with smoking or a hereditary thrombophilia).

Fekrat S, ed. *Curbside Consultation in Retina: 49 Clinical Questions, Second Edition.* (pp 41-45).
© 2019 SLACK Incorporated

Figure 8-1. "Horse." (A) Color photograph of a superotemporal branch retinal artery occlusion (BRAO) in a 78-year-old female with a Hollenhorst plaque (white arrow). (B) Fluorescein angiogram showing an occluded artery distal to the plaque.

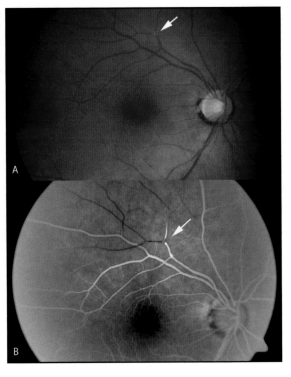

One inflammatory/autoimmune disease that should always be forefront in the mind of any clinician with an older patient with RAO is giant cell arteritis (GCA). Although less than 2% of RAOs are a result of GCA, the consequences of missing this diagnosis can be catastrophic. Therefore, unless an obvious embolus is visible on exam, I routinely order a stat erythrocyte sedimentation rate (ESR), C-reactive protein, and complete blood count (CBC) to assess platelets on all patients over age 55 with RAO, even if the patient does not have any other obvious signs or symptoms of GCA. Patients who do have a suspicious history for GCA should be started on high-dose corticosteroids immediately and referred urgently for a temporal artery biopsy. Some of the other inflammatory/autoimmune diseases that should be considered in the differential diagnosis of RAO, particularly in younger patients, are systemic lupus erythematosus, polyarteritis nodosa, granulomatosis with polyangiitis, Behcet disease, and Susac syndrome (Figure 8-2).

Traumatic causes of RAO are usually evident from the history. Inadvertent, prolonged pressure on the eye during surgery or during a drug- or alcohol-induced stupor is one cause. Patients undergoing prolonged spinal surgeries in a prone position are at particular risk for this complication. Occlusions can also be seen after retrobulbar anesthetic injections, periorbital steroid injections, and injections of cosmetic soft tissue fillers around the face.

Infectious causes of RAO are less common, but include Lyme, syphilis, tuberculosis, and toxoplasmosis.

Finally, structural abnormalities that can lead to RAO include carotid artery dissection, vasospasm during migraine, retinal arteriolar loops, and optic nerve head drusen.

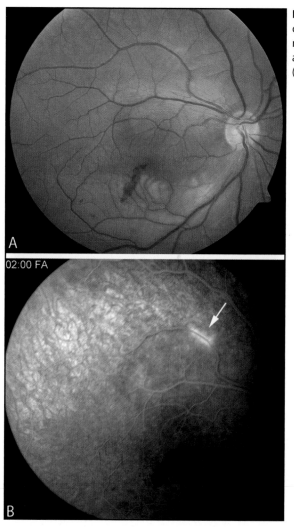

Figure 8-2. "Zebra." (A) Color photograph of an inferotemporal BRAO in a 25-year-old male with Susac syndrome. (B) Fluorescein angiogram showing focal arteriolar staining (white arrow) outside the area of occlusion.

How Do I Approach a Patient With Newly Diagnosed Branch Retinal Artery Occlusion or Central Retinal Artery Occlusion?

If a RAO is suspected to be less than 24 hours old, the first priority is to initiate urgent treatment. On optical coherence tomography, an acute RAO will show inner retinal hyper-reflectivity in the distribution of disrupted blood flow, as opposed to inner retinal thinning in a chronic RAO. For me, acute treatment includes an immediate anterior chamber paracentesis, followed by ocular massage and administration of topical aqueous suppressants. These maneuvers may help dislodge and force downstream an embolus by increasing the effective "pressure head" behind the embolus. Lowering the intraocular pressure may also help increase effective retinal perfusion pressure when the occlusion is incomplete, as is often the case. It is important to note that there is no proven benefit to these treatments; however, they are easily administered with minimal risk.

A controversial treatment option for acute management of central retinal artery occlusion (CRAO) is local intra-arterial fibrinolysis (LIF). LIF involves fluoroscopy-guided direct catheterization of the ophthalmic artery, followed by injection of recombinant tissue plasminogen activator. This is not a practical treatment for many patients with CRAO due to the constraints of time and limited availability of facilities with interventional radiologists experienced in this technique. Early studies suggested a benefit of LIF for patients who received treatment within 12 hours of symptom onset;[2] however, the more recent EAGLE (European Assessment Group for the Lysis in the Eye) study, a prospective, randomized, multicenter trial of 82 patients with acute CRAO, showed no benefit to LIF over conservative management alone at 1 month, and this study was halted early due to safety concerns (namely, a 4.5% incidence of intracranial hemorrhage in the LIF group).[3] Although LIF may still prove to be beneficial for a more limited subset of patients, the data do not support its general use currently.

Once I have administered acute treatment, I make decisions about further work-up. A fluorescein angiogram is usually not necessary to make the diagnosis, but I sometimes find it helpful in delineating a cause. Delayed or patchy choroidal filling can be seen in GCA or may indicate significant carotid or ophthalmic artery stenosis. Focal vascular staining and leakage may indicate an underlying inflammatory etiology (see Figure 8-2A). Any patient over age 55 without a visible embolus gets a stat ESR, C-reactive protein, and CBC to rule out GCA. I then refer patients to their primary care physician for further evaluation and testing.

A thorough medical history, family history, and review of systems are crucial to guiding further work-up, which can be done in a stepwise fashion. For patients over the age of 40, I generally recommend a thorough physical exam, CBC, lipid panel, carotid doppler or magnetic resonance imaging/angiogram, electrocardiogram, and transesophageal echocardiogram (with bubble study to look for septal defects). For patients under age 40, I generally recommend the same, with the exception of carotid studies. In addition, for those under age 40, I also routinely recommend fasting plasma homocysteine levels, ESR, antinuclear antibodies, antiphospholipid antibodies, and anticardiolipin antibodies.

If these initial tests fail to identify a cause for the RAO, or if something suspicious is elicited in the history or review of systems, other relevant testing might include: hemoglobin electrophoresis for sickle cell disease, Holter monitoring for arrhythmia, p-ANCA/c-ANCA for granulomatosis with polyangiitis, rheumatoid factor, FTA-ABS for latent syphilis, Lyme antibodies, Toxoplasma antibodies, PPD or Quantiferon-TB Gold assay for latent tuberculosis, or HLA-B51 for Behcet. If there is suspicion for a hereditary thrombophilia, testing should include protein C and protein S levels, antithrombin III activity, Factor V Leiden mutation, and prothrombin G20210A mutation.

Iris neovascularization occurs in 18% of CRAO patient and tends to occur earlier than in BRAO or retinal vein occlusion (as early as 2 weeks).[4] Therefore, CRAO patients may need to be seen for follow-up 2 to 3 weeks after the initial occlusion and every 3 to 4 weeks thereafter for the first 6 months to monitor for the development of iris neovascularization, neovascular glaucoma, and retinal neovascularization. Gonioscopy is recommended at these visits to monitor for neovascularization of the angle, which may precede frank iris neovascularization. The neovascularization is treated with intravitreal anti-vascular endothelial growth factor for acute control followed by sectoral (BRAO) or pan-retinal (CRAO) laser photocoagulation for long-term control.

References

1. Feinbloom D, Bauer KA. Assessment of hemostatic risk factors in predicting arterial thrombotic events. *Aterioscler Thromb Vasc Biol.* 2005;25(10):2043-2053.
2. Aldrich EM, Lee AW, Chen CS, et al. Local intraarterial fibrinolysis administered in aliquots for the treatment of central retinal artery occlusion: the Johns Hopkins Hospital experience. *Stroke.* 2008;39(6):1746-1750.
3. Schumacher M, Schmidt D, Jurklies B, et al. Central retinal artery occlusion: local intra-arterial fibrinolysis versus conservative treatment, a multicenter randomized trial. *Ophthalmology.* 2010;117(7):1367-1375.
4. Duker JS, Sivalingam A, Brown GC, Reber R. A prospective study of acute central retinal artery obstruction: the incidence of secondary ocular neovascularization. *Arch Ophthalmol.* 1991;109(3):339-342.

QUESTION

9

WHAT DO I DO WHEN I SEE A BRANCH RETINAL VEIN OCCLUSION?

Andrew M. Hendrick, MD
Michael S. Ip, MD

The diagnosis of branch retinal vein occlusion (BRVO) is made clinically. Most individuals are in their seventh decade of life and nearly two-thirds are hypertensive.[1] Other risk factors include a history of cardiovascular disease, smoking, and increased body mass. Extensive work-up following BRVO is typically not necessary in older individuals as the common risk factors are easily elicited; however, in persons under age 50 with no risk factors, a work-up may be warranted and the primary care physician consulted.

It is hypothesized that thickening of overlying branch retinal arteries within a shared adventitia results in mechanical compression of the underlying compliant venule. This occlusion of the venous circulation impairs return of blood with a spectrum of clinical findings depending on the location of the occlusion, area affected, and extent of blockage.

BRVO occurs most commonly in the superotemporal quadrant, at the junction where a branch retinal artery crosses over an underlying branch retinal vein. Sequelae of the occlusion are visible (Figure 9-1) as variable amounts of intraretinal hemorrhage, cotton-wool spots, cystoid macular edema (CME), and a tortuous dilated branch retinal vein in the affected segmental distribution distal to the site of the occluded vein. The segmental distribution is diagnostically important to distinguish BRVO from other potentially similar conditions that typically have more widespread involvement such as retinopathy from diabetes, hypertension, or radiation.

Over time, features of BRVO evolve. The intraretinal hemorrhage and any cotton-wool spots typically disappear over several weeks, although they may persist for years in some eyes. In a chronic, nonperfused BRVO, sclerosis and sheathing of the affected retinal veins may be observed. The development of venous-venous collateralization is an important feature of chronicity and provides alternative routes of venous drainage.

Fekrat S, ed. *Curbside Consultation in Retina: 49 Clinical Questions, Second Edition.* (pp 47-50).
© 2019 SLACK Incorporated

Figure 9-1. Color fundus photograph of a BRVO with intraretinal hemorrhage.

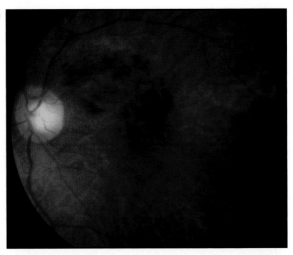

Figure 9-2. Fundus FA of a BRVO showing tortuous retinal veins and capillary dropout.

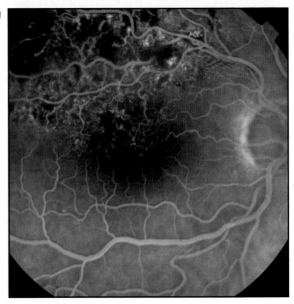

Fluorescein angiography (FA) is not mandatory to make the diagnosis of BRVO but can be useful to confirm the diagnosis and characterize the sequelae (Figure 9-2). FA often reveals a delay in venous filling within the area drained by the occluded vein, narrowed affected venous tributaries, and occasionally early hyperfluorescence just proximal to the site of occlusion. Retinal ischemia and posterior segment neovascularization are important sequelae of BRVO. FA is useful for distinguishing collateral vessels from neovascularization. Collateral vessels are flat and do not leak fluorescein in contrast to the 3-dimensionality and leakage of neovascularization. FA helps delineate the extent of capillary dropout to classify BRVO as *perfused* or *nonperfused* per the Branch Vein Occlusion Study (BVOS) criteria.[2] Although guidance from the BVOS is helpful in rendering prognosis, in clinical practice it is more useful to regard BRVO on a continuum of severity spectrum.

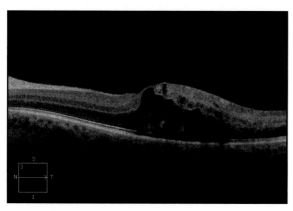

Figure 9-3. OCT, left eye. CME is present with subtle subretinal fluid.

In general, the visual prognosis of BRVO is quite favorable, but outcomes reflect disease severity. Approximately 50% to 60% of untreated eyes will have a final visual acuity of 20/40 or better. However, severe vision loss is not uncommon, with 20% to 25% resulting in visual acuity of 20/200 or worse. A final visual acuity of hand motion or worse is uncommon.[3,4]

BRVO can often be asymptomatic and does not automatically require treatment, especially if it affects areas outside the macula. In fact, therapies are directed at reversing sequelae of the impaired blood flow rather than restoring perfusion. No treatment has been established that targets eradication of the thrombosis.

CME (Figure 9-3) is the most common consequence and the leading cause of vision loss in BRVO. Optical coherence tomography (OCT) helps determine the extent of edema and monitor response to therapy. Retinal ischemia results in an increase of intraocular vascular endothelial growth factor (VEGF), which promotes breakdown of the blood retinal barrier, vascular engorgement, and CME. Historically, grid-pattern laser photocoagulation was the standard of care as demonstrated by the BVOS and is still relevant in appropriate clinical scenarios.[2] However, the BRAVO (A Study of the Efficacy and Safety of Ranibizumab Injection in Patients With Macular Edema Secondary to BRVO) and VIBRANT (Study to Assess the Clinical Efficacy and Safety of Intravitreal Aflibercept Injection in Patients With BRVO) clinical trials established the beneficial effect of intravitreal anti-VEGF medications ranibizumab and aflibercept, respectively, for CME associated with BRVO.[5,6] As a result, serial intravitreal anti-VEGF injections of ranibizumab, aflibercept, or off-label bevacizumab are now considered the standard of care. An intravitreal Ozurdex sustained-release implant (dexamethasone) is also effective at improving the CME and visual acuity as demonstrated in the GENEVA (Global Evaluation of Implantable Dexamethasone in Retinal Vein Occlusion With Macular Edema) trial.[7] Steroids have a less favorable local side effect profile due to the risk of cataract and glaucoma that temper clinical utility. Further support for this notion is found in the branch vein arm of the original SCORE (Standard Care Versus Corticosteroid for Retinal Vein Occlusion) trial. This study compared intravitreal triamcinolone to grid-pattern laser photocoagulation with similar visual outcomes, but fewer side effects were reported in the laser group.[8]

Ocular neovascularization can be a consequence of ischemic BRVO and the subsequent development of vitreous hemorrhage and rarely, neovascular glaucoma or traction retinal detachment. The risk of ocular neovascularization is between 20% to 30% and increases with larger areas of nonperfusion. These vessels are typically found at the interface of perfused and nonperfused retina. BVOS demonstrated that in eyes with retinal neovascularization, sectoral scatter laser photocoagulation reduced the risk of vitreous hemorrhage from 60% to 30%.[2] Scatter laser photocoagulation is applied with the argon green laser to achieve medium white burns (200 to 500 µm in diameter, 0.1-second duration) spaced 1 burn-width apart and covering the entire area of nonperfusion. Treatment should extend no closer than 2 disc diameters from the center of the fovea. Scatter photocoagulation targeting retinal nonperfusion preemptively is not an effective strategy for reducing CME, nor is it warranted in preventing neovascularization.

An asymptomatic BRVO that does not involve the macula can be periodically observed for neovascularization by comprehensive ophthalmologists. Consultation with a retina specialist is warranted when vision loss is present. Timing of treatment initiation is important when vision has been lost, as outcomes are better when therapy is instituted within 6 months.[5] Consultation is typically obtained within 1 to 3 weeks of BRVO diagnosis with more urgency suggested for the presence of neovascularization, vitreous hemorrhage, or traction from fibrovascular proliferation.

References

1. Klein R, Klein BE, Moss SE, Meuer SM. The epidemiology of retinal vein occlusion: the Beaver Dam Eye Study. *Trans Am Ophthalmol Soc.* 2000;98:133-41, discussion 41-43.
2. Argon laser photocoagulation for macular edema in branch vein occlusion. The Branch Vein Occlusion Study Group. *Am J Ophthalmol.* 1984;98:271-282.
3. Gutman FA, Zegarra H. The natural course of temporal retinal branch vein occlusion. *Trans Am Acad Ophthalmol Otolaryngol.* 1974;78:Op178-192.
4. Michels RG, Gass JD. The natural course of retinal branch vein obstruction. *Trans Am Acad Ophthalmol Otolaryngol.* 1974;78:Op166-177.
5. Campochiaro PA, Heier JS, Feiner L, et al. Ranibizumab for macular edema following branch retinal vein occlusion: six-month primary end point results of a phase III study. *Ophthalmology* 2010;117:1102-1112.e1.
6. Campochiaro PA, Clark WL, Boyer DS, et al. Intravitreal aflibercept for macular edema following branch retinal vein occlusion: the 24-week results of the VIBRANT study. *Ophthalmology.* 2015;122:538-544.
7. Haller JA, Bandello F, Belfort R, Jr., et al. Randomized, sham-controlled trial of dexamethasone intravitreal implant in patients with macular edema due to retinal vein occlusion. *Ophthalmology.* 2010;117:1134-46.e3.
8. Scott IU, Ip MS, VanVeldhuisen PC, et al. A randomized trial comparing the efficacy and safety of intravitreal triamcinolone with standard care to treat vision loss associated with macular Edema secondary to branch retinal vein occlusion: the Standard Care vs Corticosteroid for Retinal Vein Occlusion (SCORE) study report 6. *Arch Ophthalmol.* 2009;127:1115-1128.

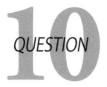

WHEN DO I REFER A PATIENT WITH A CENTRAL RETINAL VEIN OCCLUSION, WHAT IS THE WORK-UP, AND WHAT ARE THE TREATMENT OPTIONS?

Richard F. Spaide, MD

Central retinal vein occlusion (CRVO) is a condition manifested by dilated and tortuous retinal veins and intraretinal hemorrhage in all 4 quadrants of the fundus, macular edema, and variable areas of capillary nonperfusion. In the past, grading of the areas of capillary nonperfusion was used to classify eyes with CRVO into 2 distinct types based on perfusion status: (1) ischemic or nonperfused, and (2) non-ischemic or perfused.[1,2] The field of retina is one of the few in medicine in which a venous occlusion causing pathological changes is thought to be non-ischemic, highlighting the poor terminology used to describe disease. Curiously, it is not a simple matter to generate animal models that faithfully mimic CRVO. Simple ligation of the central retinal vein in primates did not produce a picture consistent with what is termed CRVO in adult humans. To produce a better approximation of the fundus picture of CRVO, simultaneous arterial occlusion had to be induced as well. Due to the lack of suitable animal models, much of what we have learned about CRVO is based on careful clinical studies of human subjects.

Patients developing CRVO note decreased vision, scotomata, and visual distortion. In the Central Vein Occlusion Study (CVOS), a collaborative study of 725 affected eyes, the baseline acuity was reported in 3 categories: (1) 29% had a good visual acuity of 20/40 or better; (2) 43% had intermediate visual acuity of 20/50 to 20/200; and (3) 28% had poor visual acuity of less than 20/200.[1] Approximately, 2/3 of patients who presented with good visual acuity maintained good visual acuity at 3 years.[1] Of those presenting with intermediate visual acuity, 19% improved to good acuity, 44% stayed in the intermediate group, and 37% decreased to poor acuity.[1] Those initially in the poor visual acuity group had an 80% chance of remaining in that group at 3 years.[1] Eyes with 10 or more disc areas of capillary nonperfusion on fluorescein angiography (FA) were

Fekrat S, ed. *Curbside Consultation in Retina: 49 Clinical Questions, Second Edition.* (pp 51-56).
© 2019 SLACK Incorporated

classified as nonperfused, while those with less than 10 disc areas were considered to be perfused. In some patients, the classification was not initially possible due to marked intraretinal hemorrhage and these eyes were termed indeterminate. Over the follow-up period, about 1/3 of eyes that were initially classified as perfused became nonperfused, while 5/6 of the eyes that were indeterminate were later classified as nonperfused. The classification of perfused vs nonperfused principally was made to predict which eyes would progress to neovascularization of the iris and angle. In the CVOS, 10% of eyes classified as perfused developed neovascularization of the iris or angle, as did 35% of the nonperfused eyes. Therefore, the classification of perfused vs nonperfused was neither very sensitive nor specific for the development of anterior segment neovascularization.

Initial treatment of decreased visual acuity in CRVO focused on macular edema. The CVOS studied the effect of grid-pattern laser photocoagulation on perfused eyes with macular edema and visual acuity of 20/50 or worse and demonstrated a beneficial anatomic effect (decreased edema on angiography), but visual acuity did not improve.[3] This study was done prior to the era of optical coherence tomography (OCT) so it is difficult to estimate the reduction in retinal thickness achieved with laser.

Subsequent therapies attempted to increase collateral vessel development because collateral vessels redirect blood flow around an area of occlusion. These therapies were largely unsuccessful, had low rates of adoption, and are now interesting historical anecdotes. They include high-power laser photocoagulation and vitreous surgical techniques for chorioretinal venous anastomosis formation and radial optic neurotomy. More recently, intravitreal injections of various pharmacologic agents have been studied in eyes with macular edema due to CRVO. Intravitreal triamcinolone[4] was associated with cataract formation, elevated intraocular pressure, and a rapid, often large, improvement in visual acuity in eyes with CRVO that was unfortunately short-lived, all of which was compounded by the need for continued injections. A randomized trial sponsored by the National Eye Institute, called the SCORE (Standard Care Versus Corticosteroid for Retinal Vein Occlusion) study, helped determine the efficacy of triamcinolone for macular edema in these eyes.

Subsequently, vascular endothelial growth factor (VEGF) inhibitors were noted to have a beneficial effect upon macular edema and visual acuity, without the risk of cataract or elevated intraocular pressure associated with triamcinolone.[5-8] We know the retina has a constitutive secretion of VEGF, and a decrease in blood flow through tissue results in an increase in VEGF production. The following are known to be true about VEGF in these eyes: (1) vitreous samples from patients with CRVO show elevated VEGF; (2) severity of CRVO is related to VEGF level; and (3) intravitreal VEGF injection in primate eyes produced findings that mimic CRVO, including venous dilation and tortuosity, intraretinal hemorrhage, telangiectasis, and areas of nonperfusion. Subsequent histopathologic analysis demonstrated endothelial cell proliferation within capillaries and venules, leading to occlusion and nonperfusion.[9] What appears to be regional nonperfusion in ischemic eyes may be the result of elevated VEGF levels, not something intrinsic to CRVO. These findings point to an alternate hypothesis implicating VEGF as an important cause of the clinical findings associated with CRVO, as opposed to simply being a sequelae of the occlusion itself.

Because VEGF may be a driving force in producing pathologic manifestations of CRVO, it is logical to use anti-VEGF agents to treat CRVO. Intravitreal Avastin (bevacizumab) was evaluated in an off-label fashion and benefits included visual acuity improvement, a decrease in macular edema, and a reduction in venous tortuosity, venous dilation, nerve swelling, and intraretinal hemorrhage in select patients. The SCORE2 study compared the efficacy of Eylea (aflibercept) with bevacizumab in eyes with CRVO.[10] The trial found that bevacizumab was non-inferior to aflibercept. A gain of at least 15 letters was reported in nearly 2/3 of the eyes and a loss of 15 letters was seen in only 2%.[10] The cost of bevacizumab is approximately 1/30 that of aflibercept, but has greater uncertainty in commercially available formulations for intraocular use and is not licensed for treatment of CRVO in some countries.

What Is the Best Way to Handle Central Retinal Vein Occlusion?

The diagnosis of CRVO is generally made by ophthalmoscopic examination and is often confirmed with FA, although this step is not necessary. FA shows that there is a slower than normal arm-to-eye time and delayed arteriovenous filling time, dilated and tortuous veins, dilated capillary segments, leakage from capillaries, staining and leakage from larger veins, and associated blocking defects from intraretinal hemorrhage. At one time, FA was a requisite test to help grade capillary nonperfusion, due to concern of the possibility of neovascular glaucoma. Today, with more mild forms of CRVO, especially when considering modern treatments, FA can be optional in some patients, provided some form of imaging documentation takes place upon diagnosis. Baseline OCT is helpful in providing an objective measurement of macular thickness and for the detection of any subretinal fluid and is used for comparison at future visits. OCT angiography (OCT-A) shows dilated and tortuous vessels with areas of capillary dilation in the superficial vascular plexus and areas of absent flow in the deep capillary plexus, particularly when there is cystoid macular edema.[11] Some patients with CRVO may also have evidence of flow problems in a cilioretinal artery, if present. Neither FA nor OCT-A shows an absence of flow in the affected ciliochoroidal vessels in these circumstances, suggesting that either the flow is rapidly restored or that diminution of flow is all that is required to induce associated ischemic retinal whitening.

Once the diagnosis is established, the next step is to consider additional testing that may be needed.[12-15] Medical work-up is not indicated for the vast majority of patients because many have well described risk factors and the results of hematologic or clotting evaluations often produce the same frequency of abnormalities as an age-adjusted normal population. Hypertension, diabetes mellitus, and glaucoma are well-known risk factors.[12-15] Referral to an appropriate specialist is indicated for patients without regular medical care, unusually severe or bilateral cases, and patients in whom a review of systems indicates other potential medical problems. Questions about past deep vein thrombosis, spontaneous abortions, or family history of clotting abnormalities may provide clues to an underlying thrombophilic disorder, but these are relatively uncommon in retinal vein occlusion patients. There are 2 common scenarios in which CRVO may be found in otherwise healthy younger individuals. The first occurs after prolonged exercise, particularly in patients who may have been dehydrated (Figure 10-1). The second is for a CRVO picture to occur in a patient with pronounced optic nerve edema. This condition has been called *thrombophlebitis*, because of a suspected associated inflammation. Indeed, inflammatory cells can sometimes be seen in the overlying vitreous by OCT.

Anti-VEGF therapy is a good first-choice treatment given the low risk of side effects and large proportion of treated patients who experience visual improvement. Choice of agents depends on the availability of a dependable source of bevacizumab and country-specific licensing. The keys to successful anti-VEGF treatment are early and repetitive treatment.[5-8] In a randomized trial, the patients assigned to delayed treatment had a worse outcome than patients treated immediately.[6,8] As there is very little risk to anti-VEGF, and conversely little gained by waiting, prompt treatment is indicated in an eye with edema and decreased visual function (Figure 10-2). I use a treat-and-extend method of administering anti-VEGF agents in eyes with CRVO. Some patients can be weaned from anti-VEGF agents, while others cannot (Figure 10-3).

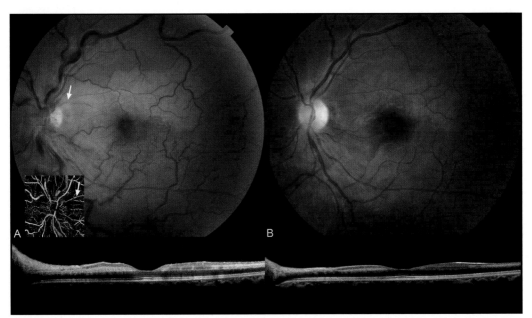

Figure 10-1. (A) This 25-year-old woman went running and then played basketball on a day when the temperature exceeded 32°C (90°F). Later, she went to sleep and, when she woke up, she had altered vision in her left eye. (Top) There are dilated and tortuous veins with some intraretinal hemorrhage. She also had an area of retinal whitening and opacification in the distribution of a cilioretinal artery (arrow). (Inset) OCT-A shows flow in the cilioretinal artery (arrow). (Bottom) The OCT through the fovea shows altered reflectivity, particularly from the inner nuclear layer. Taken in isolation, this has been referred to as *paracentral acute middle maculopathy*, a term that is somewhat misleading in that the ischemia affects more than just the middle of the macula, and it can be found outside the anatomic confines of the macula. (B) Because she had normal visual acuity and no central-involving edema, she was observed. (Top) On returning 6 weeks later, the nerve and vessels adopted a more normal appearance. (Bottom) The OCT shows some inner retinal thinning and continued opacification of the inner nuclear layer.

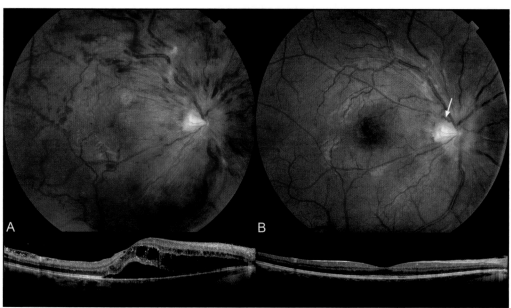

Figure 10-2. (A) (Top) The CRVO has produced typical findings of dilated and tortuous veins with a blood and thunder pattern. (Bottom) The corresponding OCT section through the fovea shows a large amount of intraretinal edema, but also subretinal fluid in the central macula. (B) (Top) After 3 intravitreal injections of an anti-VEGF agent, the patient had nearly complete resolution of intraretinal hemorrhage and much less tortuosity. There is a collateral vessel on the nerve (arrow); the presence or absence of collaterals have no significant impact on visual acuity. (Bottom) The corresponding OCT scan shows resolution of both the intraretinal edema and subretinal fluid.

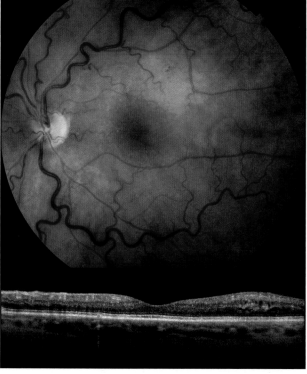

Figure 10-3. This 60-year-old had a CRVO 12 years prior, and was entered into a study using bevacizumab and then later into another trial of ranibizumab. He has been treated periodically ever since. If the interval between treatments extends past about 5 weeks, he develops marked macular edema. (Top) The retinal veins are dilated and tortuous with the blood column having a dusky hue. (Bottom) Corresponding OCT shows there is no center-involving edema, and the retinal laminae are still preserved. Receiving far more than 100 injections has been an effort, but his visual acuity is 20/30.

References

1. Central Vein Occlusion Study Group. Natural history and clinical management of central retinal vein occlusion. *Arch Ophthalmol*. 1997;115(4):486-491.
2. Central Vein Occlusion Study Group. A randomized clinical trial of early panretinal photocoagulation for ischemic central vein occlusion. Central Vein Occlusion Study Group N report. *Ophthalmology*. 1995;102(10):1434-1444.
3. Central Vein Occlusion Study Group. Evaluation of grid pattern photocoagulation for macular edema in central vein occlusion. Central Vein Occlusion Study Group M report. *Ophthalmology*. 1995;102(10):1425-1433.
4. Ip MS, Scott IU, VanVeldhuisen PC, et al. A randomized trial comparing the efficacy and safety of intravitreal triamcinolone with observation to treat vision loss associated with macular edema secondary to central retinal vein occlusion: the Standard Care vs Corticosteroid for Retinal Vein Occlusion (SCORE) study report 5. *Arch Ophthalmol*. 2009;127(9):1101-1114.
5. Spaide RF, Chang LK, Klancnik JM, et al. Prospective study of intravitreal ranibizumab as a treatment for decreased visual acuity secondary to central retinal vein occlusion. *Am J Ophthalmol*. 2009;147(2):298-306.
6. Brown DM, Campochiaro PA, Singh RP, et al. Ranibizumab for macular edema following central retinal vein occlusion: six-month primary end point results of a phase III study. *Ophthalmology*. 2010;117(6):1124-1133.e1.
7. Heier JS, Clark WL, Boyer DS, et al. Intravitreal aflibercept injection for macular edema due to central retinal vein occlusion: two-year results from the COPERNICUS study. *Ophthalmology*. 2014;121(7):1414-1420.e1.
8. Campochiaro PA, Brown DM, Awh CC, et al. Sustained benefits from ranibizumab for macular edema following central retinal vein occlusion: twelve-month outcomes of a phase III study. *Ophthalmology*. 2011;118(10):2041-2049.
9. Tolentino MJ, Miller JW, Gragoudas ES, et al. Intravitreous injections of vascular endothelial growth factor produce retinal ischemia and microangiopathy in an adult primate. *Ophthalmology*. 1996;103(11):1820-1828.
10. Scott IU, VanVeldhuisen PC, Ip MS, et al; SCORE2 Investigator Group. Effect of bevacizumab vs aflibercept on visual acuity among patients with macular edema due to central retinal vein occlusion: the SCORE2 randomized clinical trial. *JAMA*. 2017;317(20):2072-2087. doi:10.1001/JAMA.2017.4568
11. Spaide RF. Volume-rendered optical coherence tomography of retinal vein occlusion pilot study. *Am J Ophthalmol*. 2016;165:133-144.
12. The Eye Disease Case-Control Study Group. Risk factors for central retinal vein occlusion. *Arch Ophthalmol*. 1996;114(5):545-554.
13. Kolar P. Risk factors for central and branch retinal vein occlusion: a meta-analysis of published clinical data. *J Ophthalmol*. 2014;2014:724780.
14. Stem MS, Talwar N, Comer GM, Stein JD. A longitudinal analysis of risk factors associated with central retinal vein occlusion. *Ophthalmology*. 2013;120(2):362-370.
15. Sinawat S, Bunyavee C, Ratanapakorn T, et al. Systemic abnormalities associated with retinal vein occlusion in young patients. *Clin Ophthalmol*. 2017;11:441-447.

What Visualization Agents Are Used During Vitrectomy Surgery? And Wait, Tell Me About the Intraocular Tamponade Options!

Sean M. Platt, MD

Sophie J. Bakri, MD

Visualization Agents

The use of visualization agents is very popular with vitreoretinal surgeons to help visualize near-transparent tissues such as the vitreous, epiretinal membrane (ERM), internal limiting membrane (ILM), and neurosensory retina. Commonly referred to as *chromodissection*, or *chromovitrectomy* the use of different dyes can selectively accentuate the target tissue, allowing the surgeon to visualize the layer and extent of peeling. We discuss the 4 most commonly used visualization agents: triamcinolone, indocyanine green (ICG), Brilliant Blue G (BBG), and Trypan Blue (Table 11-1).

Triamcinolone acetonide (Triescence) is composed of particles in suspension, which, when injected intravitreally, are trapped within the vitreous body. This helps the surgeon visualize the vitreous itself, whether there is a posterior vitreous detachment, the boundaries of the vitreous, and an ERM when present.[1] Triamcinolone is approved for intraocular use and is not associated with retinal toxicity. Retained triamcinolone may cause elevation of intraocular pressure and should be used with caution in steroid responders or in patients with glaucoma and may contribute to cataract progression.

ICG is a popular visualization agent given its ILM selectivity and more pronounced staining effect compared to BBG (not US Food and Drug Administration [FDA]–approved, but commonly used outside the United States).[2] There is also the additional benefit of the tissue-dye interaction allowing the ILM to peel more easily, thus potentially minimizing damage to the underlying retinal layers.

Fekrat S, ed. *Curbside Consultation in Retina: 49 Clinical Questions, Second Edition.* (pp 57-60).
© 2019 SLACK Incorporated

Table 11-1
Visualization Agents Used in Vitreoretinal Surgery

Visualization Agent	Target Tissue	Concentration	Toxicity	FDA Approval
Triamcinolone	Vitreous	Variable dilutions	No, when completely removed	Yes
ICG	ILM	0.5%	Suggested	Off-label
BBG	ILM	0.025%	-	No, approved in Europe
Trypan Blue	ERM	0.15%	-	Yes

BBG also selectively stains the ILM, but not with the same intensity when compared to ICG. BBG is considered to have high biocompatibility in the eye, and thus binds well to the target tissue, is nontoxic, and degrades quickly with time. BBG is strongly absorbed at wavelengths in the visible spectrum compared to ICG, which has maximal absorption in the near infrared range. What this means is that a higher concentrations of ICG is needed compared to BBG to produce the desired effect.

Trypan Blue is used as a visualization agent to selectively stain ERM.[3] Generally, ERMs are easier to visualize under normal viewing conditions and therefore do not need to be stained. If using ICG, ILM stains but not ERM, and thus there is negative staining that identifies the ERM. However, Trypan Blue is useful in staining complex ERMs in the macula and periphery, especially those due to proliferative vitreoretinopathy (PVR), and those that seem unusually adherent. It can also help differentiate the ERM from residual posterior cortical vitreous to ensure complete removal of an ERM.

Depending on the study, dyes have been linked to toxic effects, such as visual field defects and decreased functional outcomes. Measures to limit toxicity include using a low concentration, limiting dye time in the eye, limiting peeling time, and limiting light intensity by lowering the light, and limiting exposure by moving the light pipe away from the macula.[4]

Dyes can be injected in an air- or fluid-filled eye. If you are injecting into a fluid-filled eye, you will need to mix the dye in a solution heavier than water, such as glucose or dextrose. Injecting into an air-filled eye typically results in a darker stain due to a higher effective concentration of dye.

Gas Tamponade

Using gas as an intraocular tamponade has been an important adjunct to treating retinal pathology from retinal detachments to macular holes. Many different gases are used (Table 11-2), and the choice of gas depends on the duration of tamponade desired by the surgeon.

In most instances, the gas you choose will be based on how long you need the retina approximated to the retinal pigment epithelium (RPE) for the chorioretinal adhesions to form. The force of the bubble promotes apposition of the neurosensory retina against the RPE. In eyes with a

Table 11-2
Intraocular Gases Used For
Tamponade During Vitreoretinal Surgery

Gas (Formula)	Expansion	Nonexpansile Concentration	Time to Maximum Expansion	Intraocular Duration
Air	-	-	-	3 to 5 days
Sulfur Hexafluoride (SF_6)	2x	18%	24 to 48 hours	4 to 6 weeks
Perfluoropropane (C_3F_8)	4x	14%	72 to 96 hours	6 to 8 weeks

rhegmatogenous retinal detachment, this contact is important as chorioretinal adhesions form because it keeps the retina attached and keeps fluid out of the subretinal space. The strong surface tension of a bubble allows the bubble to stay coalesced as one bubble and prevents the bubble from migrating through small retinal defects into the subretinal space.

Filtered air offers the advantage of being nonexpansile, readily available, and with the shortest longevity (3 to 5 days) among tamponade choices. Air is a great option when you do not need a long tamponade and offers a quicker visual recovery. It is the least-used gas, although it is sometimes used for pneumatic retinopexies or intraoperative retinal breaks.

Filtered air can sometimes be used in select cases of macular holes, uncomplicated retinal detachments with superior breaks, pneumatic retinopexy, and when visual recovery is needed quickly. However, for many of these cases, gas tamponade with sulfur hexafluoride (SF_6) is often chosen instead of air. More complex cases, such as retinal detachments with multiple separated breaks, inferior breaks, or PVR, may benefit from a longer-acting gas such as perfluoropropane (C_3F_8).

Silicone Oil

In cases where tamponade is needed for longer than 2 months or indefinitely, silicone oil can be used. Cases that may benefit from silicone oil tamponade include complex retinal detachments (eg, giant retinal tear, PVR, viral retinitis, traction retinal detachment due to proliferative diabetic retinopathy, traumatic retinal detachment, endophthalmitis, multiple redetachments, associated hypotony). Silicone oil is nonexpansile and will stay in the eye until it is removed surgically. It is generally left in for at least 3 months before being removed. Although silicone oil is mostly inert, it can be inflammatory and cause perisilicone oil proliferation (preretinal membranes). Other associated complications include increased intraocular pressure, cataract, corneal decompensation, subretinal oil, emulsification, unexplained vision loss, and in extremely rare cases, infiltration of the optic nerve.

There are 2 commonly used silicone oils available: lower viscosity 1000 centistokes and higher viscosity 5000 centistokes. Studies have shown no significant tamponading advantage of using a more viscous 5000 centistokes over the 1000 centistokes oil. The lower viscosity silicone oil is easier to inject and easier to remove but is associated with an increased risk of emulsification.

The choice of whether to use a longer-acting gas such as C_3F_8 or silicone oil is multifactorial[5] and is left to the surgeon's discretion.

Special Considerations for Tamponade Selection

Travel

Given the expansile nature of gases, the patient is not able to travel by air or even ground transportation where significant changes in elevation are expected while the gas bubble is present (4 weeks or more for SF_6 and 8 weeks or more for C_3F_8).

Head Positioning

Air, gas, and silicone oil all float to tamponade the retinal break; therefore, when using intraocular tamponade, it is important to position the patient's head so that the bubble apposes the retinal break. The head may be positioned looking down (for macular holes) or to the side (if there is a nasal or temporal peripheral retinal break). Many patients only need a short duration of positioning (1 to 3 days) so that the tamponade apposes the retina to the RPE to allow the cryotherapy or laser photocoagulation to take effect. Positioning can be difficult for some patients. Special equipment, such as a massage chair designed for face-down positioning, can be rented or purchased. In the presence of gas or silicone oil, the patient should be instructed not to lie on his or her back as the gas or oil may potentially hasten cataract progression and may sneak into the anterior chamber.

Visual Recovery

When air or gas is introduced into the vitreous cavity, the vision is very limited and most patients are count fingers or hand motion. Often, our surgical population may have visual limitations in the other eye so the need for a speedier visual recovery is important to maintain independence. In some eyes, selecting a tamponade with a shorter duration may be beneficial. There is an optical advantage of silicone oil because it alters the refractive error, and this may be of benefit in some monocular patients.

References

1. Peyman GA, Cheema R, Conway MD, Fang T. Triamcinolone acetonide as an aid to visualization of the vitreous and the posterior hyaloid during pars plana vitrectomy. *Retina*. 2000;20:554-555.
2. Burk SE, Da Mata AP, Snyder ME, et al. Indocyanine green-assisted peeling of the retinal internal limiting membrane. *Ophthalmology*. 2000;107:2010–2014.
3. Feron EJ, Veckeneer M, Parys-Van Ginderdeuren R, Van Lommel A, Melles GR, Stalmans P. Trypan bluestaining of epiretinal membranes in proliferative vitreoretinopathy. *Arch Ophthalmol*. 2002;120:141-144.
4. Yuen D, Gonder J, Proulx A, Liu H, Hutnik C. Comparison of the in vitro safety of intraocular dyes using two retinal cell lines: a focus on brilliant blue G and indocyanine green. *Am J Ophthalmol*. 2009;147:251-259.
5. Vitrectomy with silicone oil or perfluoropropane gas in eyes with severe proliferative vitreoretinopathy: results of a randomized clinical trial. Silicone Study Report 2. *Arch Ophthalmol*. 1992;110(6):780-792.

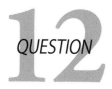

WHAT TYPE OF INTRAOCULAR LENS SHOULD BE CONSIDERED IN AN EYE WITH VITREORETINAL DISEASE?

Marina Gilca, MD

Kourous A. Rezaei, MD

It is well-documented that vitreous surgery leads to the progression of crystalline lens opacity. This is not a complication of vitrectomy surgery, but rather a pathophysiologic response to removal of the vitreous gel. The etiology of cataract formation after vitreoretinal surgery is not completely known; however, it has been reported that vitreous removal leads to increased oxygen tension in the posterior segment, resulting in oxidative damage and cataract progression.[1] We inform all of our phakic patients that they will likely need cataract surgery after vitrectomy surgery. The timing of the cataract surgery varies according to the degree of preexisting cataract, the indication for vitrectomy, the use of intraocular tamponade (type of gas bubble or silicone oil), and the patient's compliance with positioning.

Because cataract surgery is practically inevitable after vitreous surgery, we generally recommend cataract surgery prior to vitrectomy surgery for nonurgent vitreoretinal cases. This is based on the following reasons:

- Cataract surgery is generally considered easier to perform prior to vitrectomy surgery because the vitreous gel provides intraoperative support of the crystalline lens.

- If a complication develops during cataract surgery, the patient is already scheduled for vitrectomy surgery.

- An intraocular lens (IOL) generally offers a superior view during vitreous surgery when compared to an aged natural lens.

- Pseudophakic status allows for more thorough peripheral vitreous shaving.

- Inspection of the peripheral retina during vitreoretinal surgery is easier in pseudophakic eyes.

Fekrat S, ed. *Curbside Consultation in Retina: 49 Clinical Questions, Second Edition.* (pp 61-63).
© 2019 SLACK Incorporated

Our preference is to wait at least 3 weeks between cataract and vitrectomy surgery to permit the eye to quiet down and the cataract wound to heal.

There are a large variety of IOL implants currently available. The main factors that differentiate the implants are the following:

- Type of implant material: acrylic, polymethylmethacrylate, or silicone

- Hydroaffinity of the implant material: hydrophobic vs hydrophilic

- Light-filtering characteristics: blue light-filtering yellow lens vs clear lens

- Focusing characteristics: presbyopia-correcting lenses (eg, Crystalens [Bausch + Lomb], ReSTOR [Alcon Labs], Tecnis Multifocal [Abbott Medical Optics, AMO]), Symfony [AMO]) vs regular fixed-distance lenses

Polymethylmethacrylate was the first material to be used for an IOL. Current IOLs are made mainly from silicone or acrylic. In eyes with retinal pathology, cataract surgeons should avoid using silicone lenses because some complex retinal procedures may require silicone oil tamponade. Silicone oil droplets adhere irreversibly to silicone IOLs (in the presence of a posterior capsular opening), leading to a poor view of the fundus and reduced visual acuity.[2] These patients would likely need to have the IOL exchanged. This contraindication for silicone IOLs holds true for eyes with a history of silicone oil removal because silicone oil removal is never complete. The emulsified oil droplets that remain in a fluid-filled eye may adhere to the secondarily implanted silicone IOL, likely leading to reduced vision. We prefer the implantation of acrylic lenses in eyes that may need a retinal procedure in the future.

Hydrophobic IOL implants may sometimes lead to the development of glistenings: fluid-filled microvacuoles resulting from aqueous humor inflow into the IOL material.[3] Although small amounts of glistening are often unnoticed by patients and examiners, a significant amount of glistenings may occasionally impact visual acuity, contrast sensitivity, and fundus visualization during clinical exam or surgery.[4] Glistenings may worsen over time, making IOL explantation more challenging.[4] The material composition of the IOL's optic is the only currently identified risk factor for the development of glistenings.

Hydrophilic IOLs have been reported to calcify after air and/or gas exposure or breakdown of the blood-aqueous barrier and/or inflammation during intraocular surgery.[5] Some cases of IOL calcification occur only in the area that is directly exposed to air and/or gas, such as the anterior surface of IOL after Descemet stripping automated endothelial keratoplasty surgery.[6] However, IOL calcification has also been reported after uncomplicated penetrating keratoplasty or vitrectomy surgery without air/gas exposure.[7] Diabetic patients seem to have higher rates of calcification, which may be due to metabolic changes in the composition of the aqueous humor in these patients.[7,8] The Akreos Advanced Optics IOL (Bausch + Lomb), a scleral-sutured IOL, has recently become popular due to its ease of implantation and suturing; however, given its hydrophilicity, it may become calcified, and therefore may not be the optimal IOL for patients with diabetes or patients who may potentially require surgery with air or gas tamponade.[8]

We and others have reported that blue light-filtering IOLs may be beneficial in eyes that are at high risk for progression of age-related macular degeneration.[9-11] A randomized controlled clinical trial evaluated whether the yellow tint of a blue light-filtering IOL interferes with the surgeon's ability to perform vitreoretinal maneuvers.[12] Sixty patients were enrolled in this trial, and none of the surgeons reported any adverse events due to the presence of the blue light-filtering lens. No modification of the surgical set-up or procedure was required during vitreoretinal surgery.

Presbyopia-correcting IOLs currently on the market correct for both near and distance. A recent article reviewed the 2 commonly used presbyopia-correcting lenses: Crystalens and ReSTOR.[13] Crystalens is an accommodating silicone monofocal lens and is therefore contraindicated in eyes that may need vitrectomy surgery. The ReSTOR and Tecnis Multifocal are acrylic multifocal lenses and the Symfony is an extended depth of focus IOL. The accurate positioning of these lenses in the bag (single piece) or sulcus (3 piece) is crucial for its optimal performance. During vitreoretinal surgery, the eye may be filled with air or gas, which has the potential to decenter the lens from its original location. The same complication may occur in patients with toric IOLs. Multifocal and extended depth of focus lenses may induce aberrations that can interfere with intraoperative visualization of the retina. This can be especially bothersome to the vitreoretinal surgeon during membrane peeling. In addition, one may also need to refocus the microscope when operating from the posterior pole to the periphery. Patients with macular pathology therefore may not be appropriate candidates for such premium lenses. It may also be reasonable to perform optical coherence tomography in patients for whom subtle macular pathology cannot be ruled out in the setting of a significant cataract.

Summary

The selection of an appropriate IOL is important in eyes with vitreoretinal pathology. For eyes that may require vitreoretinal surgery, silicone lenses of any type should be avoided. Premium IOLs may not be suitable for patients with macular pathology.

References

1. Holekamp NM, Shui YB, Beebe DC. Vitrectomy surgery increases oxygen exposure to the lens: a possible mechanism for nuclear cataract formation. *Am J Ophthalmol.* 2005;139(2):302-310.
2. Khawly JA, Lambert RJ, Jaffe GJ. Intraocular lens changes after short- and long-term exposure to intraocular silicone oil: an in vivo study. *Ophthalmology.* 1998;105(7):1227-1233.
3. Gregori NZ, Spencer TS, Mamalis N, Olson RJ. In vitro comparison of glistening formation among hydrophobic acrylic intraocular lenses(1). *J Cataract Refract Surg.* 2002;28(7):1262-1268.
4. Christiansen G, Durcan FJ, Olson RJ, Christiansen K. Glistenings in the AcrySof intraocular lens: pilot study. *J Cataract Refract Surg.* 2001;27:728–733.
5. Neuhann IM, Neuhann TF, Rohrbach JM. Intraocular lens calcification after keratoplasty. *Cornea.* 2013;32(4):e6-10.
6. Werner L, Wilbanks G, Nieuwendaal CP, et al. Localized opacification of hydrophilic acrylic intraocular lenses after procedures using intracameral injection of air or gas. *J Cataract Refract Surg.* 2015;41(1):199-207.
7. Cao D, Zhang H, Yang C, Zhang L. Akreos Adapt AO intraocular lens opacification after vitrectomy in a diabetic patient: a case report and review of the literature. *BMC Ophthalmol.* 2016;16:82.
8. Park DH, Shin JP, Kim HK, Kim JH, Kim SY. Hydrophilic acrylic intraocular lens (Akreos AO MI60) optic opacification in patients with diabetic retinopathy. *Br J Ophthalmol.* 2010;94(12):1688-1689.
9. Sparrow JR, Miller AS, Zhou J. Blue light-absorbing intraocular lens and retinal pigment epithelium protection in vitro. *J Cataract Refract Surg.* 2004;30(4):873-878.
10. Marshall J, Cionni RJ, Davison J, et al. Clinical results of the blue-light filtering AcrySof Natural foldable acrylic intraocular lens. *J Cataract Refract Surg.* 2005;31(12):2319-2323.
11. Rezaei KA, Gasyna E, Seagle BL, Norris JR Jr, Rezaei KA. AcrySof natural filter decreases blue light-induced apoptosis in human retinal pigment epithelium. *Graefes Arch Clin Exp Ophthalmol.* 2008;246(5):671-676.
12. Falkner-Radler CI, Benesch T, Binder S. Blue light-filter intraocular lenses in vitrectomy combined with cataract surgery: results of a randomized controlled clinical trial. *Am J Ophthalmol.* 2008;145(3):499-503.
13. Tewari A, Shah GK. Presbyopia-correcting intraocular lenses: what retinal surgeons should know. *Retina.* 2008;28(4):535-537.

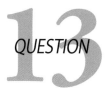

I JUST CAN'T KEEP UP WITH ALL OF THE CLINICAL TRIAL ACRONYMS. CAN YOU TELL ME WHAT STUDY EACH REFERS TO?

A. Yasin Alibhai, MD
Nadia K. Waheed, MD, MPH

Many years of clinical research have provided ophthalmologists with valuable information on natural history and treatment strategies for common retinal diseases such as age-related macular degeneration (AMD), diabetic retinopathy, and retinal vein occlusion. The introduction of intravitreal anti-vascular endothelial growth factor (anti-VEGF) injections approximately a decade ago brought about a paradigm shift in the management of some of these diseases; however, with the large number of clinical trials that have taken place in the last decade, it is often hard for the practicing ophthalmologist to keep up with the evidence base that guides our daily practice. In this chapter, we attempt to simplify and present outcomes from various landmark studies that have shaped the practice of retinal medicine as it stands today. Table 13-1 presents a summary of the clinical trials.

Fekrat S, ed. *Curbside Consultation in Retina: 49 Clinical Questions, Second Edition.* (pp 65-73).
© 2019 SLACK Incorporated

Table 13-1
Summary of Clinical Trials

Disease	Trial	Outcome
Dry AMD	AREDS1	Multivitamin formulation lowers risk of progression to advanced AMD
	AREDS2	Omega-3 of no benefit; lutein and zeaxanthin effective substitutes for beta-carotene
Wet AMD	ANCHOR and MARINA	Ranibizumab effective in treating CNV due to AMD
	PrONTO	Ranibizumab PRN dosing as effective as monthly dosing
	CATT and IVAN	Bevacizumab as effective as ranibizumab
	VIEW 1 & 2	Aflibercept as effective as ranibizumab
	SEVEN-UP	Variable visual outcomes with ranibizumab after 7 years
Diabetic Macular Edema and Diabetic Retinopathy	ETDRS	Focal laser beneficial in treating DME, aspirin ineffective in treating DR
	DRCRnet trials	**Protocol B:** Focal laser > triamcinolone for DME
		Protocol I: Ranibizumab + delayed laser most effective for DME
		Protocol T: Aflibercept, ranibizumab and bevacizumab effective for DME with ranibizumab and aflibercept more effective than bevacizumab if VA < 20/40
		Protocol S: Monthly ranibizumab as good as PRP for PDR
	RISE and RIDE	Monthly ranibizumab effective for treatment of DME
	VIVID and VISTA	Monthly and every 2 months aflibercept effective for treatment of DME
	MEAD	Intravitreal dexamethasone implant effective for treatment of DME in pseudophakic patients and phakic patients due for cataract surgery
	FAME	Intravitreal fluocinolone implant effective for treatment of persistent DME in patients previously treated with focal laser

(continued)

Table 13-1 (continued)
Summary of Clinical Trials

Disease	Trial	Outcome
Retinal Vein Occlusion	BVOS	Laser effective in treating ME due to BRVO
	CVOS	Laser ineffective in treating ME due to CRVO
	BRAVO	Ranibizumab effective in treating ME due to BRVO
	CRUISE	Ranibizumab effective in treating ME due to CRVO
	SCORE (CRVO)	Triamcinolone effective in treating ME due to CRVO
	SCORE (BRVO)	Triamcinolone as effective as laser in treating ME but associated with higher complication rate
	GALILEO and COPERNICUS	Aflibercept effective in treating ME due to CRVO
	VIBRANT	Aflibercept superior to laser in treating ME due to BRVO

PRN = as needed; PRP = panretinal laser photocoagulation; DME = diabetic macular edema; DR = diabetic retinopathy; CNV = choroidal neovascularization; VA = visual acuity; PDR = proliferative diabetic retinopathy; ME = macular edema; BRVO = branch retinal vein occlusion; CRVO = central retinal vein occlusion

Clinical Trials in Age-Related Macular Degeneration

AREDS 1 AND 2

AGE-RELATED EYE DISEASE STUDY: The AREDS studies were multicenter, randomized clinical trials that looked at the effects of antioxidants and minerals on AMD progression. AREDS1 found that people with at least intermediate AMD or with advanced AMD (geographic atrophy or macular CNV) in one eye lowered their risk of progression to advanced AMD by about 25% when treated with a high-dose combination of Vitamin C, Vitamin E, beta-carotene, and zinc.[1] AREDS2 found that omega-3 fatty acid supplementation to the original AREDS1 formulation provided no extra benefit, and that substitution of beta-carotene (associated with lung cancer in smokers) with lutein and zeaxanthin was safe and equally effective.[2]

ANCHOR AND MARINA

ANTI-VEGF ANTIBODY FOR THE TREATMENT OF PREDOMINANTLY CLASSIC CNV IN AMD AND MINIMALLY CLASSIC/OCCULT TRIAL OF THE ANTI-VEGF ANTIBODY RANIBIZUMAB IN THE TREATMENT OF NEOVASCULAR AMD: The ANCHOR and MARINA studies were 2 randomized, controlled, multicenter clinical trials that compared the efficacy of monthly intravitreal injections of the anti-VEGF drug Lucentis (ranibizumab) in the management of predominantly classic CNV and in minimally classic or occult CNV secondary to neovascular

AMD, respectively.[3,4] Patients were injected with monthly ranibizumab in the treatment arm and received photodynamic therapy (PDT) in the control arm. The ANCHOR study showed an improvement of greater than or equal to 15 letters of best-corrected visual acuity (BCVA) in up to 40% of the patients receiving ranibizumab compared to 5.6% who received PDT at 1 year. The MARINA study showed that almost 95% of patients in the ranibizumab treatment arm lost less than 15 letters at 1 year compared with 62.2% in the sham injection group. Patients receiving ranibizumab gained a mean of 7 letters compared with a loss of almost 10 letters in the control group. Consequently, ANCHOR and MARINA both proved to be landmark trials that provided strong evidence of the efficacy of ranibizumab for managing the entire spectrum of neovascular AMD.

PrONTO

Prospective OCT Imaging of Patients With Neovascular AMD: The PrONTO trial was one of the first as-needed trials in the anti-VEGF treatment of neovascular AMD. This was a prospective single center study that examined the efficacy of giving monthly intravitreal ranibizumab for the first 3 months followed by injections on an as-needed basis as determined on OCT.[5] The trial followed 40 patients with CNV secondary to neovascular AMD for 2 years with monthly clinical evaluation and OCT imaging. Following the initial 3 injections, intravitreal ranibizumab was administered based on a drop in visual acuity and/or OCT findings suggestive of CNV activity. The study found that at 1 year, 82.5% of patients maintained baseline vision and 95% lost less than 15 letters (similar to MARINA and ANCHOR). The average number of injections given at months 12 and 24 were 5.6 and 9.9, respectively. Thus, the PrONTO trial demonstrated that using an OCT-guided variable-dosing regimen meant that patients could receive fewer intravitreal injections and still achieve visual outcomes comparable to patients receiving monthly injections as had been demonstrated in ANCHOR and MARINA.

CATT and IVAN

Comparison of AMD Treatments Trials and Inhibition of VEGF in Age-Related CNV Trial: The CATT (North America) and IVAN (UK) were 2 randomized, multicenter clinical trials that compared the safety and efficacy of Avastin (bevacizumab) to that of ranibizumab in treating neovascular AMD.[6,7] They also compared individualized dosing regimen (PRN) to monthly injections. At the 1- and 2-year analysis, bevacizumab was equivalent to ranibizumab for all visual acuity outcomes when comparing monthly or PRN regimens. Fixed monthly dosing with either drug resulted in a statistically significant but clinically small improvement of about 1.5 lines of visual acuity compared with PRN dosing. Incidence of geographic atrophy development was greatest in the monthly ranibizumab group. The results of both trials provided evidence that off-label bevacizumab was an effective alternative to ranibizumab in the treatment of wet AMD at the 1- and 2-year time-points.

VIEW 1 & VIEW 2

VEGF Trap-Eye: Investigation of Efficacy and Safety in Wet AMD: VIEW 1 (North America) and VIEW 2 (rest of the world) were 2 parallel, multicenter, randomized, controlled non-inferiority clinical trials that compared monthly Eylea (aflibercept) to monthly ranibizumab in the management of neovascular AMD.[8] Both trials showed aflibercept was non-inferior to ranibizumab at maintaining visual acuity at 2 years. These results led to aflibercept gaining US Food and Drug Administration (FDA) approval.

SEVEN-UP

Seven Year Observational Update of Macular Degeneration Patients Post-MARINA/ANCHOR and HORIZON Trials: The SEVEN-UP study assessed long-term visual outcomes in patients who had participated in the ANCHOR, MARINA and HORIZON (An Open-Label Extension Trial of Ranibizumab for CNV Secondary to AMD) trials.[9] The HORIZON study was an open-label extension trial, which included patients from ANCHOR and MARINA. The study's authors reported that after a mean of 7.3 years from initially having enrolled into either ANCHOR or MARINA, only 37% of patients had a BCVA greater than or equal to 20/70. An equal number were found to have BCVA less than or equal to 20/200. These findings were attributed to undertreatment, development of fibrosis, and atrophy.

Clinical Trials in Diabetic Macular Edema and Diabetic Retinopathy

ETDRS

Early Treatment Diabetic Retinopathy Study: The ETDRS was a multicenter, randomized clinical trial designed to investigate the effectiveness of laser treatment in diabetic retinopathy. More than 3700 patients were followed for a minimum period of 4 years. The ETDRS study is of great significance because it demonstrated conclusively the benefits of focal laser photocoagulation in treating what the authors defined as *clinically significant macular edema*.[10] The study also showed that aspirin therapy had no effect on halting disease progression and that it was safe to use in patients with diabetic retinopathy who might require it for cardiovascular indications.[11]

DRCRnet

Diabetic Retinopathy Clinical Research Network: The DRCRnet is a research consortium set up in 2002 that facilitates multicenter clinical research of diabetic retinopathy, DME, and associated conditions. With more than 8500 patients enrolled in multiple protocols, it has contributed valuable research in topics ranging from follow-up using OCT, use of anti-VEGF therapy, and management of complications.

Protocol B demonstrated that intravitreal triamcinolone, when used to treat DME, had a more rapid rate of onset compared to focal laser but had poorer visual outcomes at 2 years due to a higher incidence of cataract and elevated IOP.[12]

Protocol I determined that the addition of focal/grid laser treatment at the initiation of intravitreal ranibizumab therapy for DME involving the fovea was no better, and possibly worse, for visual outcomes at 5 years compared with deferred laser treatment for ≥ 24 weeks.[13]

Protocol T showed that anti-VEGF therapy for center-involving DME using either bevacizumab, ranibizumab, or aflibercept was an effective form of treatment. For patients with visual acuity at baseline of 20/40 or better, all 3 drugs showed similar efficacy at 1 and 2 years. In patients with baseline vision of 20/50 or worse, aflibercept demonstrated statistically superior efficacy to both ranibizumab and bevacizumab at 1 year, and aflibercept and ranibizumab both demonstrated statistically similar efficacy at the 2 years, both superior to bevacizumab. All 3 drugs showed visual gains at the 2 years and a decreased need for injections, follow-up visits, and laser treatment in the second year.[14]

Protocol S reported that intravitreal ranibizumab treatment for PDR was non-inferior to panretinal laser photocoagulation at 2 years. Patients receiving monthly ranibizumab gained more letters, required fewer vitrectomies, and had lower incidences of DME.[15]

RISE AND RIDE

A STUDY OF RANIBIZUMAB INJECTION IN SUBJECTS WITH CLINICALLY SIGNIFICANT MACULAR EDEMA WITH CENTER INVOLVEMENT SECONDARY TO DIABETES MELLITUS: These were 2 identical, multicenter clinical trials that evaluated the efficacy of monthly intravitreal ranibizumab for the treatment of center-involving DME.[16] At 2 years, subjects in the 2 treatment arms of both trials reported significant gains in visual acuity (≥ 15 letters) compared to controls. Sub-analysis determined ranibizumab to be equally effective irrespective of baseline HbA1c levels. Those receiving ranibizumab were also noted to be less likely to progress to more advanced forms of diabetic retinopathy. A more recent report on the 2 trials suggested that ranibizumab slowed the progression of peripheral retinal nonperfusion in these patients with DME. The results of RISE and RIDE led to ranibizumab gaining FDA approval for the treatment of DME.

VIVID AND VISTA

INTRAVITREAL AFLIBERCEPT INJECTION IN VISION IMPAIRMENT DUE TO DME AND STUDY OF INTRAVITREAL AFLIBERCEPT INJECTION IN PATIENTS WITH DME: VIVID and VISTA were 2 identical, multicenter clinical trials that compared the efficacy of monthly and 2 monthly dosing regimens of aflibercept to macular laser therapy in treating eyes with center-involving DME.[17] For the aflibercept arm, subjects initially received monthly injections for 5 months, followed by injections either every month or every 2 months. At 2 years, subjects receiving aflibercept (either regimen) had significantly better visual outcomes and decreased central foveal thickness on OCT when compared to those receiving macular laser. The FDA only approved the every 2 months dosing schedule of aflibercept for DME treatment as the monthly regimen did not show any additional benefit.

MEAD

A STUDY OF THE SAFETY AND EFFICACY OF A NEW TREATMENT FOR DME: The MEAD study was a randomized, multicenter trial that evaluated the safety and efficacy of 0.35 mg and 0.7 mg intravitreal Ozurdex implants (dexamethasone) compared to sham injections for the treatment of DME.[18] At 3 years, patients in either of the treatment arms had significantly better visual acuity outcomes than those receiving sham injections, but the development of cataract and glaucoma was higher in the patients receiving the higher dose steroid implant. Patients in the treatment arms received an average of 4 to 5 injections over the entire 3-year period; however, those receiving steroid also had significantly higher rates of developing cataracts and elevated intraocular pressure (IOP) with around 10% in the 0.35 mg group, with less than 1% requiring glaucoma surgery. Following cataract surgery, patients had visual acuity improvements to better than baseline. As a result, the FDA-approved the Ozurdex implant for the treatment of DME, but limited its use to pseudophakic patients or in phakic patients scheduled to undergo cataract surgery.

FAME

FLUOCINOLONE ACETONIDE IN DME TRIAL: The FAME study evaluated the efficacy of long-acting intravitreal fluocinolone implants in patients with persistent DME who had previously undergone macular laser therapy.[19] After 3 years, fluocinolone showed significant improvements in visual outcomes compared with those who received sham injections. Further analysis showed that fluocinolone implants slowed diabetic retinopathy progression and delayed the onset of PDR. The rates of progression were similar to those seen with anti-VEGF treatments, but with fewer injections being required (1.3 to 1.4 injections in 3 years vs 15 to 16 injections over 2 years). However, fluocinolone implants were associated with a high incidence of cataracts (90%), elevated IOP (61%), and need for glaucoma surgery (34%).

Clinical Trials in Retinal Vein Occlusion

BVOS AND CVOS

BRANCH VEIN OCCLUSION STUDY AND CENTRAL VEIN OCCLUSION STUDY: BVOS and CVOS were randomized, multicenter trials investigating the efficacy of grid-pattern laser photocoagulation for perfused macular edema secondary to BRVO and CRVO, respectively.[20,21] The results of the BVOS showed that grid-pattern laser photocoagulation was effective in treating perfused macular edema due to BRVO; however, the CVOS results showed that visual outcomes for macular edema in eyes with CRVO treated with laser photocoagulation were not significantly different from untreated eyes.

BRAVO AND CRUISE

A STUDY OF THE EFFICACY AND SAFETY OF RANIBIZUMAB INJECTION IN PATIENTS WITH MACULAR EDEMA SECONDARY TO BRVO AND A STUDY OF THE EFFICACY AND SAFETY OF RANIBIZUMAB INJECTION IN PATIENTS WITH MACULAR EDEMA SECONDARY TO CRVO: The BRAVO and CRUISE studies were 2 Phase III clinical trials designed to investigate the efficacy and safety of ranibizumab injections in the treatment of macular edema secondary to BRVO and CRVO, respectively.[22,23] Subjects were randomized to receive either monthly ranibizumab or monthly sham injections for 12 months. Both trials showed that subjects who received ranibizumab showed a statistically significant improvement in visual acuity compared to subjects in the sham group.

SCORE

STANDARD CARE VERSUS CORTICOSTEROID FOR RETINAL VEIN OCCLUSION: The SCORE studies were 2 randomized, multicenter clinical trials designed to compare the safety and efficacy of intravitreal triamcinolone with standard of care in patients with macular edema secondary to CRVO and BRVO.[24,25] Subjects in both trials were divided into 1 of 3 groups: 2 groups received either 1 mg or 4 mg doses of triamcinolone and one group received standard clinical care (clinical observation in the CRVO trial and grid-laser in the BRVO trial). In the SCORE CRVO trial, 27% of subjects in the 1 mg group and 26% of subjects in the 4 mg group gained 15 letters or more compared with 7% in the observation only group after 12 months. In the SCORE BRVO trial, 29% of subjects in the grid-pattern laser treatment group, 26% in the 1 mg group, and 27% s in the 4 mg group gained 15 letters or more in vision at 1 year follow-up. The results of the SCORE CRVO trial were important because they showed that intravitreal triamcinolone was the first effective, long-term treatment option for CRVO patients with vision loss due to macular edema. The SCORE BRVO trial showed that while grid-laser and intravitreal triamcinolone had similar efficacy, grid-laser remains the treatment of choice in macular edema due to BRVO because of the high rates of cataract formation and elevated IOP associated with intravitreal corticosteroids.

GALILEO AND COPERNICUS

VEGF TRAP-EYE: INVESTIGATION OF EFFICACY AND SAFETY IN CRVO: These were 2 identical, randomized, multicenter trials that evaluated efficacy and safety of intravitreal aflibercept injections for treatment of macular edema secondary to CRVO.[26,27] Participants were randomized to receive either 6 monthly intravitreal injections of 2 mg aflibercept or sham injections. At the 6-month primary endpoint, 60.2% of patients in GALILEO and 56.1% in COPERNICUS receiving aflibercept gained 15 or more letters of vision compared with 22.1% and 12.3% of patients receiving sham injections, respectively. Results from both trials led to FDA approval of aflibercept treatment for macular edema secondary to CRVO.

VIBRANT

STUDY TO ASSESS THE CLINICAL EFFICACY AND SAFETY OF INTRAVITREAL AFLIBERCEPT INJECTION IN PATIENTS WITH BRVO: The VIBRANT study was a randomized, multicenter clinical trial that compared the efficacy of aflibercept with grid-pattern laser treatment in treating macular edema following BRVO.[28] In the trial, 53% of patients who received 2 mg aflibercept every 4 weeks gained at least 15 letters in vision from baseline at week 24, the primary endpoint of the study. This compared with 27% of patients in the laser treatment group who experienced similar gains in vision. Rates of serious adverse events were similar in both treatment groups (9.9% vs 9.8%). The results of VIBRANT showed aflibercept's superiority over laser treatment in treating macular edema secondary to BRVO and thus led to aflibercept gaining FDA approval for this indication.

References

1. Age-Related Eye Disease Study Research Group. A randomized, placebo-controlled, clinical trial of high-dose supplementation with vitamins C and E, beta carotene, and zinc for age-related macular degeneration and vision loss: AREDS report no. 8. *Archives Ophthalmol.* 2001;119(10):1417-1436.
2. Age-Related Eye Disease Study Research Group. A randomized, placebo-controlled, clinical trial of high-dose supplementation with vitamins C and E and beta carotene for age-related cataract and vision loss: AREDS report no. 9. *Archives Ophthalmol.* 2001;119(10):1439-1452.
3. Brown DM, Michels M, Kaiser PK, Heier JS, Sy JP, Ianchulev T. Ranibizumab versus verteporfin photodynamic therapy for neovascular age-related macular degeneration: Two-year results of the ANCHOR study. *Ophthalmology.* 2009;116(1):57-65.e55.
4. Rosenfeld PJ, Brown DM, Heier JS, et al. Ranibizumab for neovascular age-related macular degeneration. *N Engl J Med.* 2006;355(14):1419-1431.
5. Lalwani GA, Rosenfeld PJ, Fung AE, et al. A variable-dosing regimen with intravitreal ranibizumab for neovascular age-related macular degeneration: year 2 of the PrONTO Study. *Am J Ophthalmol.* 2009;148(1):43-58.e41.
6. Martin DF, Maguire MG, Fine SL, et al. Ranibizumab and bevacizumab for treatment of neovascular age-related macular degeneration: two-year results. *Ophthalmol.* 2012;119(7):1388-1398.
7. Chakravarthy U, Harding SP, Rogers CA, et al. Alternative treatments to inhibit VEGF in age-related choroidal neovascularisation: 2-year findings of the IVAN randomised controlled trial. *Lancet.* 2013;382(9900):1258-1267.
8. Heier JS, Brown DM, Chong V, et al. Intravitreal aflibercept (VEGF trap-eye) in wet age-related macular degeneration. *Ophthalmology.* 2012;119(12):2537-2548.
9. Rofagha S, Bhisitkul RB, Boyer DS, Sadda SR, Zhang K. Seven-year outcomes in ranibizumab-treated patients in ANCHOR, MARINA, and HORIZON: a multicenter cohort study (SEVEN-UP). *Ophthalmol.* 2013;120(11):2292-2299.
10. Early Treatment Diabetic Retinopathy Study Research Group. Treatment techniques and clinical guidelines for photocoagulation of diabetic macular edema. Early Treatment Diabetic Retinopathy Study Report Number 2. *Ophthalmology.* 1987;94(7):761-774.
11. Early Treatment Diabetic Retinopathy Study Research Group. Effects of aspirin treatment on diabetic retinopathy. ETDRS report number 8. *Ophthalmology.* 1991;98(5 Suppl):757-765.
12. Diabetic Retinopathy Clinical Research Network. A randomized trial comparing intravitreal triamcinolone acetonide and focal/grid photocoagulation for diabetic macular edema. *Ophthalmology.* 2008;115(9):1447-1449, 1449 e1441-1410.
13. Elman MJ, Ayala A, Bressler NM, et al. Intravitreal ranibizumab for diabetic macular edema with prompt versus deferred laser treatment: 5-year randomized trial results. *Ophthalmology.* 2015;122(2):375-381.
14. Wells JA, Glassman AR, Ayala AR, et al. Aflibercept, bevacizumab, or ranibizumab for diabetic macular edema: two-year results from a comparative effectiveness randomized clinical trial. *Ophthalmology.* 2016;123(6):1351-1359.
15. Gross JG, Glassman AR, et al; Writing Committee for the Diabetic Retinopathy Clinical Research Network. Panretinal photocoagulation vs intravitreous ranibizumab for proliferative diabetic retinopathy: a randomized clinical trial. *JAMA.* 2015;314(20):2137-2146.
16. Nguyen QD, Brown DM, Marcus DM, et al. Ranibizumab for diabetic macular edema: results from 2 phase III randomized trials: RISE and RIDE. *Ophthalmology.* 2012;119(4):789-801.

17. Korobelnik JF, Do DV, Schmidt-Erfurth U, et al. Intravitreal aflibercept for diabetic macular edema. *Ophthalmology*. 2014;121(11):2247-2254.

18. Boyer DS, Yoon YH, Belfort R, Jr., et al. Three-year, randomized, sham-controlled trial of dexamethasone intravitreal implant in patients with diabetic macular edema. *Ophthalmology*. 2014;121(10):1904-1914.

19. Campochiaro PA, Brown DM, Pearson A, et al. Long-term benefit of sustained-delivery fluocinolone acetonide vitreous inserts for diabetic macular edema. *Ophthalmology*. 2011;118(4):626-635.e622.

20. Branch Vein Occlusion Study Group. Argon laser photocoagulation for macular edema in branch vein occlusion. *Am J Ophthalmol*. 1984;98(3):271-282.

21. Central Vein Occlusion Study Group. Evaluation of grid pattern photocoagulation for macular edema in central vein occlusion. The Central Vein Occlusion Study Group M report. *Ophthalmology*. 1995;102(10):1425-1433.

22. Brown DM, Campochiaro PA, Bhisitkul RB, et al. Sustained benefits from ranibizumab for macular edema following branch retinal vein occlusion: 12-month outcomes of a phase III study. *Ophthalmology*. 2011;118(8):1594-1602.

23. Brown DM, Campochiaro PA, Singh RP, et al. Ranibizumab for macular edema following central retinal vein occlusion: six-month primary end point results of a phase III study. *Ophthalmology*. 2010;117(6):1124-1133.e1121.

24. Ip MS, Scott IU, VanVeldhuisen PC, et al; SCORE Study Research Group. A randomized trial comparing the efficacy and safety of intravitreal triamcinolone with observation to treat vision loss associated with macular edema secondary to central retinal vein occlusion: the Standard Care vs Corticosteroid for Retinal Vein Occlusion (SCORE) study report 5. *Archives Ophthalmol*. 2009;127(9):1101-1114.

25. Scott IU, Ip MS, VanVeldhuisen PC, et al; SCORE Study Research Group. A randomized trial comparing the efficacy and safety of intravitreal triamcinolone with standard care to treat vision loss associated with macular edema secondary to branch retinal vein occlusion: the Standard Care vs Corticosteroid for Retinal Vein Occlusion (SCORE) study report 6. *Arch Ophtahlmol*. 2009;127(9):1115-1128.

26. Korobelnik JF, Holz FG, Roider J, et al. Intravitreal aflibercept injection for macular edema resulting from central retinal vein occlusion: one-year results of the phase 3 GALILEO Study. *Ophthalmology*. 2014;121(1):202-208.

27. Heier JS, Clark WL, Boyer DS, et al. Intravitreal aflibercept injection for macular edema due to central retinal vein occlusion: two-year results from the COPERNICUS study. *Ophthalmology*. 2014;121(7):1414-1420.e1411.

28. Clark WL, Boyer DS, Heier JS, et al. Intravitreal Aflibercept for Macular Edema Following Branch Retinal Vein Occlusion: 52-Week Results of the VIBRANT Study. *Ophthalmology*. 2016;123(2):330-336.

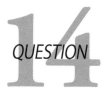

QUESTION

14

HOW DO I FIGURE OUT WHETHER OR NOT MY PATIENT HAS A POSTERIOR VITREOUS DETACHMENT? DOES THERE HAVE TO BE A WEISS RING TO MAKE THE DIAGNOSIS?

Stephen G. Schwartz, MD, MBA
Harry W. Flynn, Jr., MD
Ingrid U. Scott, MD, MPH

Posterior vitreous detachment (PVD) is a common age-related event that may be associated with multiple vision-threatening retinal conditions, including retinal break, rhegmatogenous retinal detachment (RRD), vitreomacular interface disorders, proliferative diabetic retinopathy (PDR) in persons with diabetes, and others.[1] Interestingly, this common and important finding lacks a clinically validated diagnostic endpoint. The Weiss ring (Figure 14-1) traditionally has been considered a specific sign of a completed PVD, in the sense that a patient with an ophthalmoscopically visible Weiss ring is thought to have a PVD.[2]

The Weiss ring, however, is not a definitive sign of a PVD, and some eyes with PVD do not have a Weiss ring.[3] For example, in one series of 200 eyes with a PVD diagnosed using biomicroscopy, the authors reported a complete Weiss ring in 51%, an incomplete Weiss ring in 36%, and no Weiss ring in 13%.[4]

B-scan echography (Figure 14-2) may be a more sensitive test for PVD than biomicroscopy. The Phase III Microplasmin for Intravitreous Injection–Traction Release Without Surgical Treatment clinical trial specified the use of B-scan "to evaluate the status of the posterior vitreous cortex."[5] More recently, swept source optical coherence tomography (OCT) has been reported to image the posterior vitreous cortex and differentiate partial from complete PVD.[6]

The use of ancillary testing to diagnose PVD in routine clinical care is variable. Some authors report that ultrasonography is routinely used to diagnose or confirm PVD,[7] but we tend not to use this technique (or OCT) frequently in clinical practice for the purpose of diagnosing or confirming PVD. Typically, a PVD is documented if a complete or partial Weiss ring can be determined by biomicroscopy, and vitreous syneresis or possible PVD is used to describe the status of the vitreous in which a Weiss ring is not detected.

Fekrat S, ed. *Curbside Consultation in Retina: 49 Clinical Questions, Second Edition.* (pp 75-78).

Figure 14-1. Color fundus photograph, left eye, demonstrating a broken Weiss ring in a patient with a complete PVD.

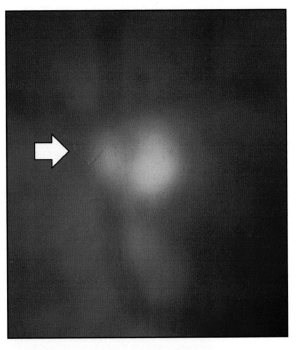

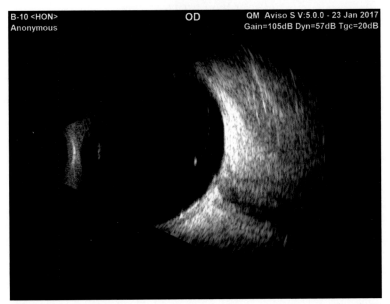

Figure 14-2. B-scan echography, right eye, demonstrating a complete PVD. The area of increased signal along the posterior hyaloid represents the Weiss ring.

Therefore, the short answers to the questions, "How do I figure out whether or not my patient has a PVD?" and "Does there have to be a Weiss ring to diagnose the diagnosis?" are "with clinical examination and, optionally, B-scan echography or OCT" and "no." Perhaps an additional question at this juncture is, "Does it matter?"

During pars plana vitrectomy (PPV), induction of a PVD in an eye with an attached posterior hyaloid may be an important step in the surgery. In one series of 96 eyes with high myopia that underwent PPV, intraoperative diagnosis (usually with staining agents) of complete PVD was made in 52% of eyes, and the finding of PVD was significantly associated with the preoperative diagnosis. Specifically, PVD was noted in 85% of eyes with RRD and 74% with epiretinal membrane, but only 14% of eyes with myopic foveal schisis and 10% with macular hole.[8]

Outside the context of PPV, does the definitive diagnosis of a PVD affect clinical management decisions? In the very common situation of a patient with new-onset or worsening complaints of flashes or floaters, we suggest that the clinical management (in this case, dilated fundus examination including scleral depression as needed) is the same regardless of the presence or absence of a PVD.

The status of the posterior vitreous may be important in the pathogenesis of certain retinal diseases. It has been taught traditionally that vitreomacular traction (VMT) is important in the development of full-thickness macular hole,[9] but some macular holes occur months or years following documented release of VMT[10] or PPV for RRD.[11] Similarly, it has been taught traditionally that retinal neovascularization in PDR grows along the scaffold of the posterior hyaloid.[12] To that effect, a Phase II randomized clinical trial evaluating the use of ocriplasmin to induce a PVD in an attempt to reduce the development of PDR is currently recruiting patients.[13] However, a case of recurrent PDR with 2 areas of neovascularization elsewhere has been reported in an eye with a complete PVD, determined by the presence of a Weiss ring and confirmed using B-scan echography and OCT.[14] Thus, a PVD does not guarantee that a patient will not subsequently develop a macular hole or PDR in that eye.

The relationship between PVD and response to anti-vascular endothelial growth factor (anti-VEGF) treatment for neovascular age-related macular degeneration (AMD) is unknown. In one retrospective series of 61 eyes treated with anti-VEGF agents, the presence of PVD was determined using B-scan echography, and patients with and without PVD were compared. Presence of a PVD was associated with significantly larger visual acuity improvement, but not with greater reduction in OCT-measured central subfield thickness.[15] In one prospective series of 93 patients treated with anti-VEGF therapy for neovascular AMD, the presence of PVD was not significantly associated with the magnitude of visual acuity improvement nor with magnitude of central subfield thickness reduction on OCT.[16]

Clinicians strive to perform the best clinical examination that they can. A definitive answer to the question "Does my patient have a PVD?" may be very important in a research setting, a prospective clinical trial, or a patient being considered for PPV. For the vast majority of patients, however, this question may not affect subsequent clinical management. The presence of a PVD traditionally has suggested a lower risk of future PDR, RRD, macular hole, and other conditions, although the presence of a PVD does not prevent any of these entities and, in our opinion, treatment recommendations and follow-up intervals are generally not affected by the presence or absence of a Weiss ring.

References

1. Johnson MW. Posterior vitreous detachment: evolution and complications of its early stages. *Am J Ophthalmol.* 2010;149(3):371-382.
2. De Bustros S. Vitrectomy for prevention of macular holes. Results of a randomized multicenter clinical trial. Vitrectomy for Prevention of Macular Hole Study Group. *Ophthalmology.* 1994;101(6):1055-1059.
3. Murakami K, Jalkh AE, Avila MP, Trempe CL, Schepens CL. Vitreous floaters. *Ophthalmology.* 1983;90(11):1271-1276.
4. Kakehashi A, Inoda S, Shimizu Y, Makino S, Shimizu H. Predictive value of floaters in the diagnosis of posterior vitreous detachment. *Am J Ophthalmol.* 1998;125(1):113-115.
5. Stalmans P, Benz MS, Gandorfer A, et al. Enzymatic vitreolysis with ocriplasmin for vitreomacular traction and macular holes. *N Engl J Med.* 2012;367(7):606-615.
6. Bertelmann T, Goos C, Sekundo W, Schulze S, Mennel S. Is optical coherence tomography a useful tool to objectively detect actual posterior vitreous adhesion status? *Case Rep Ophthalmol Med.* 2016;2016:3953147.

Table 15-1

Suggested Guidelines for Triaging Patients With Floaters

1. Create a triage template that prompts staff to ask pertinent questions and record pertinent positive and negative symptoms and history.
2. Checklist for pertinent symptoms:
   - ☐ New onset floaters or a change or worsening of chronic floaters
   - ☐ Duration of floaters
   - ☐ Associated symptoms (ie, photopsias, decreased central vision, and peripheral vision loss)
   - ☐ History of prior retinal breaks or detachments in the symptomatic eye and fellow eye
   - ☐ Family history of retinal detachment
   - ☐ History of trauma in the symptomatic eye
   - ☐ Type(s) and date(s) of prior ocular surgery (including yttrium-aluminum-garnet capsulotomy) in the symptomatic eye
   - ☐ Pain, redness, or photophobia, which may indicate uveitis, including endophthalmitis, in a patient who has had recent eye surgery or systemic illness
   - ☐ History of systemic conditions that may predispose to problems that cause floaters (eg, diabetes with vitreous hemorrhage, AIDS with potential for cytomegalovirus retinitis, collagen vascular disease with the potential for uveitis)
3. In general, patients with new onset floaters of less than 2 weeks duration should be instructed to come within 24 hours, preferably the same day. This is especially true if the patient has associated symptoms of photopsia, central or peripheral vision loss, ocular pain, redness, photophobia, history of recent eye surgery or trauma, history of a systemic condition that could predispose to vitreous hemorrhage, intraocular infection, or noninfectious intraocular inflammation.
4. Patients with subacute floaters (> 2 weeks but < 6 weeks) without associated photopsias; central or peripheral vision loss; and no pain, redness, or photophobia should be told to come in within 1 week and should call back and come in the same day if photopsias, vision loss, pain, redness, or photophobia develop before the scheduled appointment.
5. Patients with floaters of more than 6 weeks duration are more difficult to triage.
   a. In general, if floaters are worsening or if there is associated central or peripheral vision loss, photopsias, or a systemic condition with the potential for infection, hemorrhage, or inflammation, the patient should be told to come in the same day.
   b. Evaluation of chronic floaters with no associated symptoms or underlying systemic condition of concern can be scheduled within 1 month with instructions to call back before the scheduled appointment if symptoms worsen or new concerning symptoms (reviewed with the patient in lay terms) develop.

Evaluation

A complete ocular and systemic history and ocular examination with dilation of both eyes should be performed so that causes of floaters other than posterior vitreous detachment (PVD) are not overlooked. In our practice, we have provided guidelines for the pertinent information to be recorded, and we have instructed technicians and house staff to discuss pertinent abnormalities with an attending physician before dilation. The following are the key examination findings to be recorded:

- Current refraction and corrected distance and near visual acuity of each eye with pinhole testing for distance. If pinhole visual acuity is not 20/20, then I ask that a diagnostic refraction be attempted. If this information is not recorded at the first visit, it is easy to overlook later. If a patient subsequently requires retinal detachment repair, knowledge of his or her preoperative visual acuity and refraction allows me to counsel him or her about visual prognosis and potential postoperative refractive changes.

- Visual fields by confrontation to document visual field loss (or lack thereof).

- Pupil size and reaction to light and testing for an afferent pupillary defect (or documentation that the patient presented with the pupils already dilated). Note that if only one eye is dilated, the presence or absence of an afferent defect can be detected by reverse testing.

- Basic ocular motility examination. While formal motility testing with prisms is not usually performed in the setting of acute PVD symptoms, any preexisting ocular misalignment in primary gaze or limited motility should be documented. Such findings could subsequently become important should the patient require retinal detachment repair.

- Slit-lamp examination. Both undilated (when possible) and dilated slit lamp examination should be performed. Record media opacities, signs of current or past intraocular inflammation, trauma, or surgery, iris abnormalities, lens status, posterior capsule status, and presence or absence of anterior vitreous cells or pigment.

- Dilated ophthalmoscopic examination. I typically examine the posterior pole with slit-lamp biomicroscopy and a 90 diopters (D) lens first. I then inspect the entire fundus with binocular indirect ophthalmoscopy and scleral indentation of the peripheral retina for 360° using a 20 D lens (or 28 D lens for small pupils). This is sufficient for most patients; however, if I have not found a break by that point but still suspect a break based on symptoms or other findings, I perform a contact lens examination using a Goldmann 3-mirror fundus lens (Volk). I record the presence or absence of a Weiss ring and the location of all retinal pathology in relation to vascular and other landmarks.

Ancillary Testing

If the entire fundus cannot be visualized because of media opacity, a small pupil, or a patient's inability to cooperate, I perform B-scan ultrasonography of the entire posterior segment. A carefully performed ultrasound can detect even a small peripheral retinal detachment or tear and can detect the presence and extent of a PVD and any associated vitreoretinal traction.

Optical coherence tomography (OCT) can help identify early PVD and can determine whether the fovea is detached in the setting of a shallow macular detachment or mild media opacity. In one case diagnosed as a macula-off retinal detachment because of poor vision and poor visualization of the macula, OCT demonstrated that the central macula was attached and that the decreased vision was due to a focal vitreous hemorrhage overlying the central macula.

"Why so many questions?" you may ask. Well, many of the white dot syndromes can look similar, and a detailed history will help us determine if this disease is a local ocular process or part of a systemic inflammatory disease. Also, asking these questions can help assess whether further work-up is needed. It also ensures that potential infectious masquerades are not missed, particularly tuberculosis and syphilis.

Armed with this information, a complete examination is needed to determine the location, severity, and chronicity of inflammation. We quantitate the severity of inflammatory cell and flare and look for signs of previous inflammation, such as posterior synechiae, keratic precipitates, and pigment on the lens. Nodules on the iris and/or conjunctiva can point to diseases such as sarcoidosis, tuberculosis, or even lymphoma.

When examining the posterior segment, we quantify the amount of vitreous inflammation and look at the size, color, and characteristics of the white dots. Are they small (less than the caliber of the central retinal artery), large (bigger than the optic nerve), or in between? Are they round or irregular? Are the borders sharp or ill-defined? Are the dots white or yellow, atrophic-appearing or pigmented (this helps to determine the level of activity)? Is there any associated hemorrhage or vascular sheathing? Finally, we look for any changes around the optic nerve, such as edema, peripapillary atrophy, or tilting.

Imaging is vital in this disease category, as it will unmask the location of lesions and assist in determining disease activity. Once we determine which imaging test reveals the disease activity particularly well, we then use that imaging test to follow the patient. Ultra-widefield fluorescein angiography and widefield indocyanine green angiography assist in identifying the location of choroidal and retina lesions, especially in the periphery. Additionally, angiography can differentiate between inactive and active areas. Usually, active areas will block early and hyperfluoresce late and have indistinct borders, while inactive borders tend to either hypofluoresce or stain and have sharp borders. Indocyanine green angiography can assist in identifying choroidal lesions that are not readily seen.

Optical coherence tomography (OCT) is important as it provides crucial cross-sectional information. Imaging of the macula and of suspicious lesions outside the macula should be obtained. OCT assists in determining the location of inflammation, the level of activity based on the disruption of the outer retinal structures. Furthermore, OCT can identify cystoid macular edema, intra- or subretinal fluid, the latter raising concern for secondary choroidal neovascularization (CNV). OCT is also useful in visualizing choroidal structures.

Additional imaging tests, such as fundus autofluorescence and OCT angiography (OCT-A), are obtained in certain situations. Fundus autofluorescence can be useful in identifying active lesions which typically hyperautofluoresce. OCT-A is useful in identifying CNV and assessing vascular perfusion, as well as identifying flow voids or abnormalities corresponding to choroidal lesions.

Armed with the information from the history, examination, and imaging, it is now time to develop a differential. It is important to remember that many of these diseases are idiopathic in origin and have overlapping features. It is vital not to miss an infectious etiology and crucial to identify features that may imply a systemic disease or masquerade. We first determine the location, chronicity, and severity of inflammation. In patients with panuveitis, we begin with diseases such as multifocal choroiditis, sarcoidosis, syphilis, tuberculosis, and rarely lymphoma. We use the imaging findings to help us further. Choroidal involvement implies sarcoidosis and tuberculosis, while broad, plaque-like changes in the outer retina is suspicious for syphilis. Large subretinal lesions would be concerning for lymphoma.

In those diseases with posterior involvement, we use the size of the lesions and imaging findings to further categorize them. Smaller dots are suspicious for diseases such as multiple evanescent white dot syndrome, punctate inner choroidopathy (PIC), and multifocal choroiditis (MFC). PIC and MFC lesions tend to be punched out when inactive and have gray/white borders when active. Multiple evanescent white dot syndrome lesions are typically very small and are often missed, but identified on imaging. Syphilis, sarcoidosis, and tuberculosis can masquerade as any of these smaller lesion diseases. Diseases such as birdshot choroidopathy and lymphoma can also mimic the appearance of some of these smaller dots, especially with MFC involvement.

More confluent, larger, or placoid lesions point toward conditions like acute posterior multifocal placoid pigment epitheliopathy or serpiginous chorioretinitis. When active, these diseases have characteristic fluorescein angiographic features, including blocking early and hyperfluorescing late. Still, syphilis, sarcoidosis, and tuberculosis are often included in the differential for these larger lesion diseases.

Ultimately, some of these may be difficult to distinguish definitively at the first visit, but we try to develop a strong suspicion for infectious vs inflammatory conditions. At the initial visit, we will test for infectious diseases, such as syphilis and tuberculosis, and based on the findings and differential, inflammatory diseases, such as sarcoidosis. Once we have ruled out infectious etiologies, corticosteroids can be used to treat active inflammation, especially in those with vision threatening diseases such as MFC, serpiginous, and PIC. Although controversial, we will often treat acute posterior multifocal placoid pigment epitheliopathy patients with systemic corticosteroids to speed recovery and limit permanent damage. Imaging is used to follow these patients to monitor response to therapy. In those with more chronic disease, systemic immune suppression is needed to control the disease. Secondary complications, such as CNV, are treated with local anti-vascular endothelial growth factor therapy.

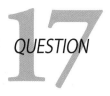

HOW DO I WORK UP AND MANAGE A PATIENT WITH A WHITE-CENTERED RETINAL HEMORRHAGE?

Seema Garg, MD, PhD

Although originally thought to be pathognomonic for subacute bacterial endocarditis (SBE), a white-centered retinal hemorrhage (WCRH), often called a *Roth spot*,[1] is seen in a variety of systemic and ocular conditions.

While the pathologic basis of the white centers may be focal ischemia, inflammatory infiltrate, a colony of infectious organisms, or accumulation of neoplastic cells, most often it is a fibrin-platelet plug.[2] In the latter case, the plug forms in response to acute retinal capillary rupture. While the myriad causes of WCRH may seem unrelated, most of them show a common predisposition to capillary extravasation. The WCRH is actually a manifestation of the capillary bleeding and subsequent repair process.

One way to think about the differential of WCRH is to determine the mechanism of capillary rupture.[3,4] For instance, thrombocytopenia (resulting from low-grade disseminated intravascular coagulopathy from SBE or leukemia) can cause capillary bleeding. Furthermore, ischemia from other causes (eg, anemia, anoxia, carbon monoxide poisoning, prolonged intubation) can cause damage to the retinal capillary endothelium, and resultant bleeding. Increased capillary fragility (seen in diseases such as hypertension, preeclampsia, and diabetes) can also cause capillary rupture. Elevated venous pressure (seen in intracranial hemorrhage, birth trauma, and nonaccidental injury in infants) can also be the cause of capillary rupture. Thus, keeping in mind the mechanism of capillary rupture helps to understand the diverse causes of the WCRH.

I have divided diseases associated with WCRH into disorders of the hematopoietic system, immune-mediated collagen vascular disease, trauma, disseminated fungal or bacterial infection, ischemia (including ocular ischemic syndrome [OIS] and preeclampsia), and vascular malformations. Less often, WCRH can be seen in patients with diabetes mellitus but usually only if there is an acute change in blood glucose.

Fekrat S, ed. *Curbside Consultation in Retina: 49 Clinical Questions, Second Edition.* (pp 87-90).
© 2019 SLACK Incorporated

Figure 17-1. Right fundus of asymptomatic 47-year-old with multiple scattered white-centered retinal hemorrhages.

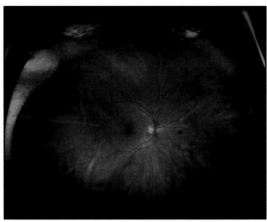

Work-Up

So, how does one differentiate between all these seemingly disparate causes of a WCRH? The first step is a thorough patient history, review of systems, and ophthalmoscopic examination. Based on ocular findings, as well as certain systemic examination findings, the appropriate laboratory work-up can be initiated.

If a patient has a disorder of the hematopoietic system, such as anemia,[5] leukemia,[6] or multiple myeloma,[7] a thorough history may reveal that the patient has a preexisting acute or chronic hematologic disorder. If the patient is anemic, he or she may have symptoms, such as fatigue or shortness of breath on exertion. The patient may have signs of thrombocytopenia, such as petechiae. In addition to WCRH, the ocular exam may reveal a hypopyon, disc edema, retinal vascular sheathing, and cotton-wool spots in cases of leukemia. A laboratory work-up should consist of a complete blood count, which would be abnormal in anemia and leukemia (leukocytosis and thrombocytopenia). At this point, it would be important to consult with a hematologist/oncologist, who may note immature abnormal white blood cells in the peripheral smear as well as on a bone marrow biopsy. Figure 17-1 shows fundus photos of a completely asymptomatic 47-year-old healthy male in which WCRH hemorrhages were noted incidentally. After a thorough history revealed no preexisting conditions and a negative review of systems, a complete blood count showed leukocytosis (white blood cell count = 108,000/mcL, normal range 3500 to 10,000/mcL). The patient was immediately referred to the hematologist/oncologist who performed a bone marrow biopsy and ultimately diagnosed chronic myelogenous leukemia (CML). The importance of the role of ophthalmologist in the diagnosis of asymptomatic individuals cannot be underestimated. In this case, the presence of WCRH and a high index of suspicion by the ophthalmologist led to the appropriate work-up and diagnosis of leukemia.

If a patient has an immune-mediated collagen vascular disease, such as polyarteritis nodosa, a history may reveal muscle and joint pain, excessive fatigue, and abdominal pain. In addition to WCRH, the ocular exam may show uveitis, scleritis, and retinal vascular sheathing. Laboratory work-up for immune-mediated collagen vascular diseases would include an erythrocyte sedimentation rate, C-reactive protein, antinuclear antibodies, rheumatoid factor, antineutrophil cytoplasmic antibodies, and complement factors, and, if abnormal, consultation with a rheumatologist for further work up and management.

Disseminated fungal, viral, or bacterial infections can cause WCRH, as in cases of fungemia, syphilis, HIV, or ocular toxoplasmosis.[8] The exam may show cell or flare in the anterior chamber, posterior uveitis, or even panuveitis. The work-up should include an aqueous or vitreous tap, a serum rapid plasma reagin/fluorescent treponemal antibody-absorption to rule out syphilis and

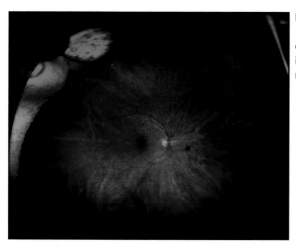

Figure 17-2. Right fundus of same patient 1 month after treatment with imatinib, an oral cancer treatment for CML. Note marked improvement of scattered white-centered retinal hemorrhages.

a serum HIV test. With a history of a recent fever and new heart murmur, consider serial blood cultures as well as a transesophageal echocardiogram to evaluate for valve vegetations in cases of suspected SBE.

If a patient has a history of trauma, resulting in intracranial hemorrhage, WCRH may be seen. Infants can present with WCRH due to birth trauma, but nonaccidental injury should be considered, especially if accompanied by intracranial hemorrhage and/or bone fractures. Patients can develop WCRH after intracranial hemorrhage from arteriovenous malformation or aneurysm. Symptoms may include headache and vision changes and warrant head imaging with either computed tomography, magnetic resonance imaging, or magnetic resonance angiography.

Patients with a history of cardiovascular disease may have OIS. If you suspect OIS and note WCRH, obtain carotid doppler ultrasonography. In the event of significant carotid stenosis, the patient may be a candidate for carotid endarterectomy.

WCRH is less commonly found with hypertension and diabetic mellitus, but can occur if there is an acute change in blood glucose or uncontrolled blood pressure. In a study of eyes with varying levels of diabetic retinopathy, 15.6% had at least 1 WCRH and less than 5% showed 5 or more WCRHs.[9] In addition to WCRH, one would expect to find other typical changes of diabetic retinopathy such as microaneurysms, dot-blot hemorrhages, hard exudates, and cotton-wool spots. The laboratory work-up would include a serum glucose (> 140 mg/L), HbA1c (> 6.5%), and urinalysis (glycosuria and ketonuria).

If you suspect undiagnosed hypertension, obtain a HbA1c and blood pressure reading, respectively.

If a pregnant patient has WCRH and vision loss, consider the diagnosis of early preeclampsia and refer for obstetric assessment.[10]

Management

As the etiologies are so varied, many of the causes of WCRH require comanagement with our physician colleagues from a variety of subspecialties, as described previously after the initial management. In most cases, after treating the underlying systemic cause, WCRH will resolve. Visually, they are asymptomatic unless the macula is involved, so there is no ophthalmologic management of the WCRH itself. Figure 17-2 shows nearly complete resolution of the WCRH after only 1 month of treatment with imatinib, an oral cancer treatment for CML.

Summary

The diagnostic strategy for WCRH includes a detailed patient history, a complete review of systems, a thorough ophthalmologic examination, followed by targeted testing to rule out the various associated systemic conditions. Determining the etiology can be truly lifesaving.

References

1. Litten M. Ueber akute maligne Endocarditis und die dabei vorkommended retinal veranderungne. *Charite-Ann.* 1878;3:137-190.
2. Duane TD, Osher RH, Green WR. White centered hemorrhages: their significance. *Ophthalmology.* 1980;87(1):66-69.
3. Pomeranz HD. Roth spots. *Arch Ophthalmol.* 2002;120(11):1596.
4. Ling R, James B. White-centred retinal hemorrhages (Roth spots). *Postgrad Med J.* 1998;(74):581-582.
5. Zehetner C., Bechrakis N. E. White centered retinal hemorrhages in vitamin B12 deficiency anemia. *Case Rep Ophthalmol.* 2011;2(2):140–144.
6. Lepore FE. Roth's spots in leukemic retinopathy. *N Engl J Med.* 1995;332:5:335.
7. Priluck JC, Chalam KV and Grover S. Spectral-domain optical coherence tomography of Roth spots in multiple myeloma. *Eye (Lond).* 2012;26(12):1588–1589.
8. Furtado JM, Toscano M, Castro V, Rodrigues MW. Roth spots in ocular toxoplasmosis. *Ocul Immunol Inflamm.* 206;24(5):568-570.
9. Catalano RA, Tanenbaum HL, Majerovics A, Brassel T, Kassoff A. White centered retinal hemorrhages in DR. *Ophthalmology.* 1987;94:388-92.
10. Capoor S, Goble RR, Wheatley T, Casswell AG. White-centered retinal hemorrhages as an early sign of preeclampsia. *Am J of Ophthalmology.* 1995;119(6):804-806.

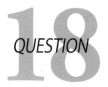

HOW DO I MANAGE A SUPRACHOROIDAL HEMORRHAGE?

Odette Margit Houghton, MD

Nicholas Farber, MD

A suprachoroidal hemorrhage (SCH) is a potentially devastating complication of intraocular surgery caused by rupture of the posterior ciliary arteries. Though commonly associated with anterior segment surgery, it can occur with any intraocular procedure. SCHs are typically stratified as acute, with occurrence during the procedure, or as a postoperative complication. Risk factors thought to be associated with SCH include advanced age, previous pars plana vitrectomy, history of elevated intraocular pressure (IOP) and/or glaucoma, increased axial length, and atherosclerosis.[1]

The key to preserving an eye with an acute intraoperative SCH is early recognition and prompt action prior to the expulsion of intraocular contents. Acknowledge and prepare yourself for the possibility prior to every intraocular surgical procedure and craft a management strategy in advance in order to have all of the necessary tools immediately available.

Early signs of a SCH include eye pain; increased posterior pressure; loss of the red reflex; enlargement of the pupil; shallowing of the anterior chamber with forward displacement of the iris, lens, or lens implant; and vitreous prolapse. If a SCH is suspected, all surgical wounds should be closed immediately. The purpose is to elevate the IOP sufficiently to tamponade the suprachoroidal bleeding. Ideally, close the wound with 8-0 sutures. If there is no time to place sutures, approximate the wound edges with digital pressure or toothed forceps. Wound closure is much faster with preplaced sutures and well-constructed incisions. If you have a penetrating keratoplasty incision, close the globe with a temporary keratoprosthesis.

The risk of vitreous incarceration may be reduced with maintenance or reformation of the anterior chamber with saline or air, but a highly cohesive viscoelastic substance is usually required. Tissue incarceration is usually best managed during a secondary procedure. However, if you are convinced the hemorrhage is limited and there is no further bleeding, then reopening, cleaning, and closing small sections of the wound in sequence may be considered, but is not generally recommended.[2]

Fekrat S, ed. *Curbside Consultation in Retina: 49 Clinical Questions, Second Edition.* (pp 91-94).
© 2019 SLACK Incorporated

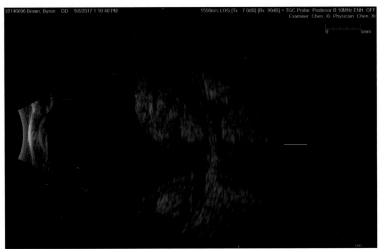

Figure 18-1. B-scan ultrasound showing choroidal detachment with hyperechogenic suprachoroidal material, indicating likely hemorrhage.

If extrusion of intraocular contents limits the ability to close all wounds, external drainage via sclerotomies may be necessary to reposition the tissue; however, primary drainage is hazardous and should be avoided if possible. Acute drainage could reverse the tamponade effect of the secondarily elevated IOP and result in additional suprachoroidal bleeding. Conversely, drainage may be unsuccessful due to the extremely fast clotting of a SCH, usually before an emergency sclerotomy can even be performed. Following external drainage, if performed, the sclerotomies should be sutured closed, and the anterior chamber should be reformed, if possible.

Most limited intraoperative and delayed postoperative choroidal hemorrhages resolve with observation within weeks to a few months. They should be followed with serial echography to monitor for apposition and liquefaction (Figure 18-1). Appositional, or *kissing*, hemorrhagic choroidals are thought to have a worse prognosis. A case-control study from the Cleveland Clinic showed no difference in outcomes with observation vs surgery in this appositional group.[1] During the postoperative period, topical and oral prednisone (1 mg/kg/day) is recommended to control inflammation and reduce the likelihood of intraocular tissue adhesion. Elevated IOP requires aggressive topical, and sometimes oral, therapy. Eye pain due to stretching of the posterior ciliary nerves can be managed with topical cycloplegia and oral analgesia.

With nonappositional detachments, not all patients benefit from a secondary procedure. Indications for surgical management and choroidal drainage include development of central retinal apposition that does not resolve within 1 to 2 weeks, shallow/flat anterior chamber with secondary IOP elevation, hypotony, persistent flat anterior chamber, or intractable eye pain. First address any causes of hypotony, such as wound leak, shallow retinal detachment, or ciliary body detachment. Drainage may need to be combined with a vitrectomy if there is rhegmatogenous or tractional retinal detachment, incarceration of intraocular tissues, retained lens material, vitreous hemorrhage, or extensive subretinal hemorrhage.

An SCH is easier to drain after 10 to 14 days because the clotted blood has a greater chance of being liquefied. Recombinant tissue plasminogen activator injected into the suprachoroidal space has been used to enhance liquefaction prior to surgery.[3] Echographic characteristics of liquefaction include reduced reflectivity on A-scan and a more echolucent pattern on B-scan.[4] Many surgeons believe that the optimal drainage location is the highest point of choroidal elevation, as determined by echography or ophthalmoscopy. Good exposure of the drainage site can usually be achieved with a conjunctival peritomy, followed by isolation of a rectus muscle with a silk tie or

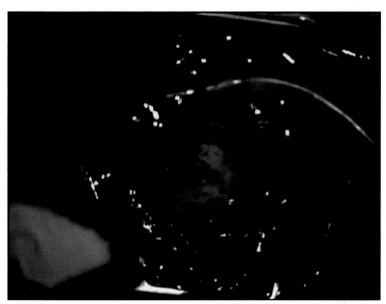

Figure 18-2. Intraoperative photo during drainage of a suprachoroidal hemorrhage. A 6-0 silk traction suture is utilized for exposure and an anterior chamber infusion maintains consistent IOP. A radial cutdown is being performed, making sure to be at least 6 mm posterior to the limbus.

placement of a scleral traction suture. Drainage sclerotomies should be radial and created with a cut-down incision, at least 6 mm posterior to the limbus (Figure 18-2). Alternatively, an anterior sclerotomy created in a similar fashion as for pars plana vitreous surgery may be used. More than one sclerotomy may be required in opposite quadrants. Drainage can be promoted by manipulating the sclerotomy with forceps, cotton-tip applicators, or a cyclodialysis spatula within the wound. Alternatively, 6-0 traction sutures can be placed on the wound edge. Active aspiration under direct visualization using a guarded 26-gauge needle attached to the extrusion line from the vitrectomy console has also been described.[5]

Throughout the drainage procedure, the IOP must be maintained with an intraocular infusion. In order to reduce the risk of iatrogenic damage to the anteriorly displaced retina, the infusion can be introduced through the limbus via a 23-gauge needle, a small gauge vitrectomy infusion cannula, or an anterior chamber maintainer. Alternatively, some surgeons prefer to render the patient aphakic and use an anterior limbal approach or 6 mm infusion cannula to ensure entry into the vitreous cavity. Establish the infusion prior to placement of the sclerotomies to avoid hypotony. Precise IOP is difficult to maintain using a syringe or gravity infusion. A constant intraocular infusion pressure (preset between 20 mmHg and 30 mmHg) is easier to maintain with a continuous pressurized infusion system.[6]

The standard intraocular infusion commonly used is balanced saline solution. If there is adequate communication between the anterior and posterior chambers, viscoelastic or air can be utilized. When vitreoretinal surgery is anticipated, the choice of substitute is limited to clear liquids. Perfluorocarbon liquid is particularly useful as a primary substitute or as an adjunct in this instance. Perfluorocarbon liquid displaces vitreous, lens fragments, and suprachoroidal and subretinal hemorrhage anteriorly. When using perfluorocarbon liquids, placing the sclerotomies anterior to the equator may assist drainage of the SCH.[7]

Once normal anatomic configuration of the pars plana has been reestablished with drainage, a conventional 3-port pars plana arrangement can be performed. If there is vitreous or retinal incarceration before or during drainage, anterior vitrectomy through the limbus or pars plana should be considered prior to further drainage. Once drainage is complete, the retina may need to be delaminated from anterior structures. A relaxing retinotomy or scleral buckle may be required for residual vitreoretinal traction. A nonexpansile long-acting gas such as 14% C_3F_8 can be used for internal tamponade. You may prefer to use silicone oil in eyes in the following situations:

- Large relaxing retinotomies
- High risk of proliferative vitreoretinopathy
- Hypotony
- Recurrent SCH

If you use silicone oil, be aware that after resolution of the SCH, the silicone oil fill may be insufficient.

Any residual choroidal hemorrhage remaining after drainage should completely resolve over a few weeks to months, similar to nonappositional suprachoroidal detachments under observation. Eyes should be monitored for postoperative complications, such as hypotony, retinal detachment, proliferative vitreoretinopathy, persistent pain, and even phthisis.

References

1. Moshfeghi DM, Kim BY, Kaiser PK, et al. Appositional suprachoroidal hemorrhage: a case- control study. *Am J Ophth*. 2004;13 (6):959-963.
2. Kuhn F, Morris R, Mester V. Choroidal detachment and expulsive choroidal hemorrhage. *Ophthalmol Clin North Am*. 2001;14(4):639-650.
3. Kunjukunju N, Gonzales CR, Rodden WS. Recombinant tissue plasminogen activator in the treatment of supra-choroidal hemorrhage. *Clinical Ophthalmology*. 2011;5:155-157.
4. Chu TG, Green RL. Suprachoroidal hemorrhage. *Surv Ophthalmol*. 1999;43(6):471-486.
5. Mandelcorn ED, Kitchens JW, , Fijalkowski N, Moshfeghi DM. Active Aspiration of suprachoroidal hemorrhage using a guarded needle. *Ophthal Surgery, Lasers & Imaging Retina*. 2014;45(2):150-152.
6. Lakhanpal V, Schocket SS, Elman MJ, Nirankari VS. A new modified vitreoretinal surgical approach in the management of massive suprachoroidal hemorrhage. *Ophthalmology*. 1989;96(6):793-800.
7. Desai UR, Peyman GA, Chen CJ, et al. Use of perfluoroperhydrophenanthrene in the management of suprachoroidal hemorrhages. *Ophthalmol*. 1992;99(10):1542-1547.

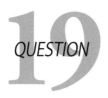

WHEN SHOULD I SUSPECT ENDOPHTHALMITIS IN MY POSTOPERATIVE CATARACT PATIENT AND WHAT ARE THE TREATMENT OPTIONS?

Bernard H. Doft, MD

Post–cataract surgery endophthalmitis is one of the most dreaded complications of cataract surgery. The incidence may be rising in correspondence with increased use of clear corneal surgery, and it could be as high as 2 to 3/1000 operations. Recent data based on multicenter trials suggests that prophylactic intracameral antibiotics may markedly decrease the rate of post-cataract endophthalmitis. All cataract surgeons should become familiar with this data and make a decision whether or not to employ this approach. However, the topic of this review is not prophylaxis, but rather about diagnosis and treatment. Every ophthalmologist recognizes the typical case of a patient presenting a few days after surgery with a painful red eye, count fingers vision, a hypopyon, and a limited view posteriorly; however, there are much more subtle presentations, and early detection can result in better outcomes. Making an early diagnosis can sometimes be difficult. When should you suspect endophthalmitis? Once you suspect it, what do you do? To address these questions, let us look at a few patients presenting at various time points after cataract surgery.

Patient 1 comes in on the first postoperative day. He has a bit of discomfort. Vision is 20/60. At the slit-lamp, you see mild corneal edema and a definite hypopyon. When you look behind the intraocular lens (IOL), the vitreous is clear. Is this endophthalmitis? It can be hard to tell. If endophthalmitis is presenting this early, such as on the first postoperative day, it is likely due to a pretty virulent organism, yet the vitreous in this patient is clear. Does that make sense? What do you do? The answer is watch the patient for a few hours and have another look. Okay, so it doesn't get worse in those few hours. What now? Well, it still could be endophthalmitis, but more likely you need to think about toxic anterior segment syndrome (TASS). Watch a bit longer, and look

Fekrat S, ed. *Curbside Consultation in Retina: 49 Clinical Questions, Second Edition.* (pp 95-98).
© 2019 SLACK Incorporated

Figure 19-1. Classic postoperative endophthalmitis with hypopyon. Fibrin strands are present.

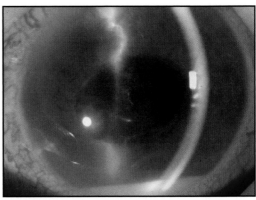

again in a few more hours. If the vitreous remains quiet, then it is probably TASS. This syndrome is not infectious endophthalmitis, and management is entirely different than for endophthalmitis.

Patient 2 comes in on the first postoperative day, just like Patient 1. You had performed clear corneal cataract extraction with posterior chamber IOL insertion. After the patient arrives, you wait a few hours and look again. The hypopyon is bigger, and there is fibrin in the anterior chamber (AC), and the vitreous is becoming cloudy. The patient became worse in those few hours. Now you have your diagnosis. Endophthalmitis that presents this early is probably due to a virulent organism, causing the rapid increase in inflammation. Emergency treatment is necessary.

Let us look at Patient 3. It is 5 to 6 days postoperatively. The patient comes in for a routine exam. She has no complaints but states, "My vision isn't perfect, Doc." On exam, vision is 20/50, the cornea is clear, the IOL is in good position, and with a careful exam, you see definite cells in the AC but no hypopyon. It is a bit more inflammation than you are used to seeing, and there are also some cells in the vitreous. "My surgery went well," you say. "Why should there be a cellular reaction in the AC?" Keep asking yourself that question. Do not let the absence of pain or the absence of a hypopyon fool you. Perform gonioscopy. There are times that one can see a small layering of cells in the inferior angle with a gonioscopy lens when one cannot really appreciate it at the slit-lamp alone. Remember, you don't have to have a hypopyon to diagnose endophthalmitis. This is another patient to watch carefully. See the patient several hours later. If things are getting worse when you see the patient later that day, there is a good chance it is endophthalmitis. It is probably better to err on the side of over diagnosis in this case, even if you are not yet positive that there is an infection.

Okay, now let's look at Patient 4. It is 3 to 5 days after surgery. The patient says, "My eye aches." Of course, your staff had the patient come right over. On exam, visual acuity is 20/800, and the eye is red. The AC shows a 1-mm layered hypopyon, cells, and fibrin strands (Figure 19-1). The vitreous is cloudy. With indirect ophthalmoscopy, you can just barely make out the retina. No mystery here! This is classic postoperative endophthalmitis.

Now, here's a variant. Patient 5 presents just like Patient 4 except he is diabetic. Management might differ, so read on.

One more patient is Patient 6. He has the exact same presentation as Patient 4 except that vision on presentation is light perception (LP) only. He cannot appreciate hand motion. The diagnosis is obvious endophthalmitis as in Patients 4, 5, and 6, and the presentations are textbook. Treatment options vary depending on presentation, so read the following.

Here is our last patient, Patient 7. It is more than 6 weeks since his surgery, but it can even be a year or longer. The patient came in a month early for his checkup. He has mild complaints about blurred vision in the eye in question. Acuity is 20/40. The eye looks white. There is no hypopyon, but there is a mild AC reaction with a few keratic precipitates (Figure 19-2). You see some creamy

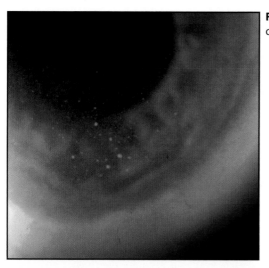

Figure 19-2. Keratic precipitates in an eye with chronic indolent endophthalmitis.

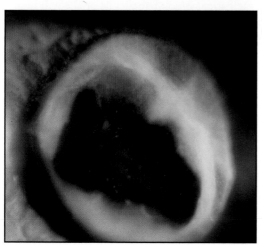

Figure 19-3. Creamy white opacifications of the capsule in chronic indolent endophthalmitis.

opacification of the posterior capsule. (Things can get to the point that this capsular opacification is much worse, as shown in Figure 19-3). The vitreous has some inflammation that might look like a small string of pearls, but it is mild. The eye appears to have mild uveitis. Most likely, the diagnosis is chronic indolent endophthalmitis. Management is quite different than for patients who present with more acute endophthalmitis.

Well, you have made your diagnosis, or at least you are suspicious enough to consider it. Here are a few points. If you are a cataract surgeon, and if you even think of acute postoperative endophthalmitis, and I mean even think of it, assume that is what it is until proven otherwise. It is much safer for your patient if you proceed that way. I have often had cataract surgeons call me and say, "I saw this patient yesterday morning, and the eye looked inflamed, so I increased the frequency of topical antibiotics and steroids. Today it is much worse." Remember, endophthalmitis should never be treated with topical medications alone. If you are thinking infection, refer the patient to a retinal specialist. Using increased frequency of topical drops will just cause you to lose valuable time. If the eye is infected, it will only get worse, and you will have delayed appropriate treatment. So, when in doubt, send it out! (That is, send it to your local retina specialist for another opinion.)

What Are the Treatment Options?

Okay, the diagnosis is made. Let's go patient by patient. First, Patient 1. The patient presented on the first postoperative day with a hypopyon, but clear vitreous, and did not progress to have vitreous involvement with observation. This patient with TASS does not have endophthalmitis. There is no space to deal with management of TASS here, but it involves treating with steroids, controlling pressure, corneal edema, etc. Look it up if you are not familiar with this syndrome.

Patients 2, 3, and 4 are all managed in the same way. Each is a patient with acute post-cataract surgery endophthalmitis presenting with vision of counting fingers or better. Standard of care treatment involves obtaining cultures of the aqueous or vitreous, injection of intravitreal antibiotics, and prescribing postoperative topical antibiotics. Time is of the essence. Depending on the patient's drug allergies, intravitreal antibiotics include intravitreal vancomycin 1 mg in 0.1 cc, and either amikacin 0.4 mg in 0.1 cc or ceftazidime 2 mg in 0.1 cc. Vitrectomy is usually not required when patients present with hand motion or better vision, as visual outcomes with intravitreal injection are similar to outcomes with vitrectomy. Refer this patient out immediately, do not wait until the next day. If your retinal specialist is not immediately available, find another one! The patient can probably be managed as an outpatient, and if the patient is not diabetic, he or she will have a better than 60% chance of ending up 20/40 or better.

Patient 5 is a bit different, as he is diabetic. Based on published data, your patient may have a better outcome if a vitrectomy is performed, as opposed to just a tap and injection of antibiotics alone, even if vision is hand motion or better.

In Patient 6, the presenting vision is LP only. There is unequivocal randomized trial data which shows that when post-cataract extraction patients present with endophthalmitis and LP only vision, a vitrectomy is required, and your patient should have one immediately. Even with this severe presentation, outcomes can be excellent with one-third of eyes achieving a visual acuity of 20/40 or better.

Our last patient, Patient 7, most likely has chronic indolent endophthalmitis. This is not an emergency. Depending on presentation, if you are not sure of the diagnosis, you might want to treat this patient with topical steroids and watch. Sometimes things will get better, but then relapse. When it does, it is time to refer this patient out for definitive treatment. The low virulence organisms are often sequestered in the lens capsule. Management options vary, but often the best outcomes will occur with vitrectomy, intravitreal antibiotics, capsulectomy, and lens exchange or removal.

Suggested Reading

Doft BH, Wisniewski SR, Kelsey SF, Fitzgerald SG; Endophthalmitis Vitrectomy Study Group. Diabetes and postoperative endophthalmitis in the endophthalmitis vitrectomy study. *Arch Ophthalmol.* 2001;119(5):650-656.

Endophthalmitis Vitrectomy Study Group. Results of the Endophthalmitis Vitrectomy Study: a randomized trial of immediate vitrectomy and of intravenous antibiotics for the treatment of postoperative bacterial endophthalmitis. *Arch Ophthalmol.* 1995;113(12):1479-1496.

Javitt JC. Intracameral antibiotics reduce the risk of endophthalmitis after cataract surgery: does the preponderance of the evidence mandate a global change in practice. *Ophthalmology.* 2016;123:226-231

Mamalis N, Edelhauser HF, Dawson DG, Chew J, LeBoyer RM, Werner L. Toxic anterior segment syndrome. *J Cataract Refract Surg.* 2006;32(2):324-333.

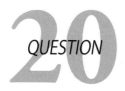

HOW DO I FOLLOW A PATIENT WITH A PRESUMED CHOROIDAL NEVUS?

Matthew A. Powers, MD, MBA

Prithvi Mruthyunjaya, MD, MHS

Choroidal melanocytic proliferations produce a range of clinical manifestations that include benign, premalignant, and malignant conditions. As the vast majority of these lesions are defined by their clinical features, and less commonly by a confirmatory biopsy, there can be some controversy and confusion over how to characterize and follow a particular lesion.

In our ocular oncology clinic, lesions are divided into 3 broad categories: (1) benign (low suspicion for malignancy), (2) indeterminate (medium to high suspicion for malignancy), and (3) malignant. To determine which category a lesion belongs in, we combine patient history with clinical examination, ancillary imaging studies, and standardized ultrasonography. The clinical challenge is to define reliable parameters for a particular benign or premalignant lesion that make it more or less likely to progress into a malignancy.

A benign choroidal nevus (BCN) is a common finding in the adult White population, although only 1/9000 will progress into malignant uveal melanoma (UM). BCN are typically minimally elevated, brown in color (but may be variably pigmented), and have a base between 1 and 10 mm and an apical height of less than 1.5 mm.[1] In addition, BCN are characterized by a smooth surface and sometimes possess overlying drusen and retinal pigment epithelium (RPE) disruption, features which are often indications of chronicity (Figure 20-1). BCN can still exhibit normal growth at a slow rate, which should not be confused with malignant transformation. Less common but still benign conditions include choroidal melanocytosis, which is caused by hyperplasia of melanocytes and characterized by patchy areas of flat choroidal pigmentation, and choroidal freckle, which is caused by increased melanin without hyperplasia and presents as a flat pigmented lesion less than 2 disc diameters that remains stationary over time.

Fekrat S, ed. *Curbside Consultation in Retina: 49 Clinical Questions, Second Edition.* (pp 99-104).
© 2019 SLACK Incorporated

Figure 20-1. Choroidal nevus with overlying drusen, estimated to have a low risk for growth or malignant transformation.

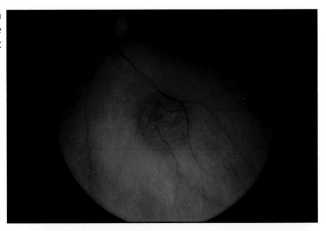

Figure 20-2. ICL with moderate risk of growth and progression into a UM. Specifically, this demonstrates pigmented nevus with a more posterior location and subretinal fluid.

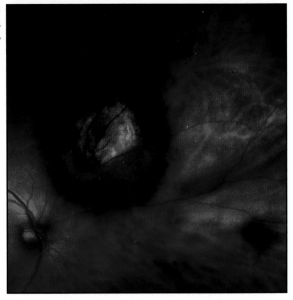

The more concerning lesion is what we refer to as an *indeterminate choroidal lesion* (ICL), sometimes called *atypical* or *suspicious choroidal nevus*. These are not definitively UM, but may exhibit one or more clinical features that historically are associated with an active UM. The presence of these features may represent risk factors for future growth and progression to malignant UM.

We specifically ask patients if they are having any visual symptoms that may suggest fluid exudation or lesion growth (eg, photopsias, visual field changes) and if they are, then we aggressively seek out any prior fundus photos to compare previous documentation of the lesion, including evidence of change or growth of the lesion.

Key clinical examination features to note include pigmentation pattern (predominantly melanotic, amelanotic, or mixed pigmentation), an estimate of the size and distance to the fovea and optic nerve (in millimeters or disc diameters), the presence of subretinal fluid (SRF) (eg, overlying or adjacent to the lesion), lipofuscin accumulation, characterized by orange pigment, presence of drusen, or associated RPE alterations near the lesion, indicative of previous SRF (also referred to as *high water mark*) (Figure 20-2). All lesions are photographed and optical coherence tomography (OCT) images of the lesion are obtained. A standard 10 MHz B-scan ultrasound probe is used to

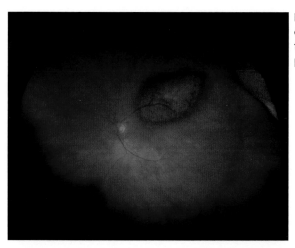

Figure 20-3. Widefield scanning laser ophthalmoscopy image clearly demonstrates the anatomical context of a large, posterior, pigmented lesion.

measure the lesion's base and height. This baseline information is vital in formulating an accurate diagnosis and planning for future follow-up.

Multimodal ophthalmic imaging is an invaluable tool in the diagnosis and monitoring of these lesions. In general, we rely on standard and widefield fundus photography, ultrasonography, spectral domain OCT (SD-OCT), and fundus autofluorescence (FAF). Recently, OCT angiography has also emerged as a new technology and will likely be an important component of tumor imaging in the future, although at present, its benefits are still being investigated. Separately, each of these can help discern important prognostic features of choroidal lesions.

Fundus photography is essential to document all margins of the tumor, as well as provide a reference view of the proximal macula and optic nerve (Figure 20-3). Widefield imaging provides panoramic views of a lesion but may not accurately document lesion color. Whereas standard fundus photography reliably documents lesion color, it may require multiple images to construct a montage large enough to see all lesion borders. Regardless, all lesions should be photographed.

Using scanning laser ophthalmoscopy, FAF helps identify the presence of possible lipofuscin in the RPE, a product of normal aging and oxidative damage, but which is also found in active UMs. Hypoautofluorescence overlying choroidal lesions is suggestive of chronic RPE damage and suggests possible tumor inactivity and chronicity. Hyperautofluorescence, on the other hand, is associated with acute damage to the RPE and accumulation of lipofuscin granules and may suggest a high-risk lesion (Figure 20-4).[2]

SD-OCT is an important tool to diagnose and monitor suspicious choroidal lesions. High-density scans over the lesion surface provides excellent ultrastructural information and can provide evidence of both choroidal and retinal morphological changes. SD-OCT it can detect drusen more accurately or confirm the presence of lipofuscin. It can also detect photoreceptor loss, ellipsoid zone irregularity, RPE atrophy, or pigment epithelial detachment, all signs of chronicity.

Importantly, OCT may help distinguish between intraretinal cystic fluid accumulation, so-called *subclinical microedema*, typically a sign of chronicity, and active neurosensory retinal separation from SRF, typically a sign of an active lesion. It is important to note, however, that SRF at the apex of the lesion, rather than the base, is associated with chronicity and a more favorable prognosis. Early studies have demonstrated an association between active basal SRF on OCT and subsequent growth of ICLs, suggesting that such a finding must be monitored very closely.[3]

Figure 20-4. FAF image demonstrating speckled hyperautofluorescence overlying a choroidal tumor, a finding indicating accumulation of lipofuscin, which conveys a high risk of malignancy.

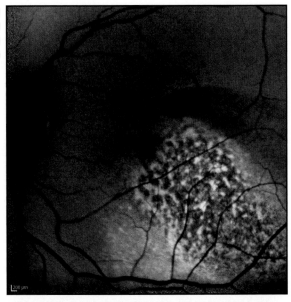

Figure 20-5. OCT over a lesion demonstrates neurosensory retinal detachment with subretinal fluid and irregular-appearing photoreceptors, a sign associated with subsequent growth.

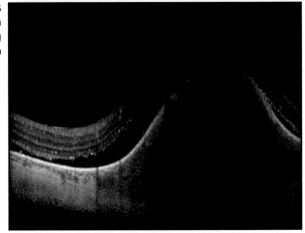

Enhanced depth imaging (EDI)-OCT involves focusing the OCT device further posterior into the choroid and may provide more information about suspicious lesions than standard OCT. On studies of EDI imaging, choroidal nevi have demonstrated choriocapillaris compression and overlying RPE atrophy. Choroidal melanomas, on the other hand, demonstrate increased choroidal thickness, deep optical shadowing, and fresh overlying subretinal fluid with shaggy-appearing photoreceptors (Figure 20-5).[4]

Swept source OCT (SS-OCT) is another new OCT modality, which uses a longer wavelength (1050 nm vs 850 nm), allowing for deeper penetration of light and the ability to image more posterior structures. SS-OCT appears to be superior to SD-OCT in terms of imaging intralesional details. In addition, SS-OCT imaging of choroidal nevi has demonstrated the presence of a hyporeflective band separating the tumor from the RPE, most likely representing the choriocapillaris. Benign nevi on SS-OCT still often display a partial or complete shadowing of deeper structures, but in the absence of shadowing, the choroidoscleral junction can sometimes be visualized below the lesion. Finally, in choroidal nevi, the suprachoroidal layer and suprachoroidal space is often visible in close proximity to the lesion.[5]

Table 20-1
Risk Factors for Growth of a Small Indeterminate Choroidal Lesion

- Thickness (≥2 mm)
- Proximity to the optic nerve (≤3 mm)
- Presence of subretinal fluid
- Presence of orange pigment
- Presence of visual symptoms
- Absence of drusen

EDI may be close to replacing ultrasonography in select thinner lesions for measuring tumor thickness, because ultrasound may overestimate tumor thickness. This is because ultrasound measures both the retinal and choroidal components of the lesion. OCT has been able to successfully quantify tumor thickness in about half of all tested lesions, but with greater accuracy in very small lesions due to its higher resolution than ultrasound. However, current OCT technology limits measurable tumors to those under 2.5-mm thick due to its inability to clearly resolve the choroidoscleral junction.[6]

Retrospective studies have identified several exam features at presentation that may help predict growth of a small ICL into a UM. See Table 20-1 for a list of features.[7,8] Risk stratification suggests that patients with ICLs associated with more than one of these features should be counseled as to the significant chance of growth over a 5-year period.[8] Such lesions require very close follow-up or, preferably, an evaluation by an ocular oncologist.

Careful follow-up is important with any lesion. The presence of even the most benign-appearing lesion should be conveyed to the patient and his or her primary ophthalmologist to ensure yearly follow-up. We monitor medium- to high-suspicion ICLs at least every 4 months for 1 year and, if completely stable, may subsequently extend the interval to every 6 months. In the case of a highly suspicious ICL or a small melanoma that the patient elects not to have treated, reevaluations are conducted no longer than 3 months apart or sooner if new visual symptoms are reported.

Any evidence of growth or the development of new features that arise during the course of routine follow-up, such as expansion of lesion borders, new subretinal fluid, or change in ultrasound characteristics, should prompt further evaluation by an ocular oncologist.

References

1. Augsburger JJ, Corrêa ZM, Trichopoulos N, Shaikh A. Size overlap between benign melanocytic choroidal nevi and choroidal malignant melanoma. *Invest Ophthalmol Vis Sci.* 2008;49(7):2823-2828.
2. Almeida A, Kaliki S, Shields CL. Autofluorescence of intraocular tumours. *Curr Opin Ophthalmol.* 2013;24(3):222-232.
3. Espinoza G, Rosenblatt, Harbour JW. Optical coherence tomography in the evaluation of retinal changes associated with suspicious choroidal melanocytic tumors. *Am J Ophthalmol.* 2004;137(1):90-95.

4. Shah SU, Kaliki S, Shields CL, Ferenczy SR, Harmon SA, Shields JA. Enhanced depth imaging optical coherence tomography of choroidal nevus in 104 cases. *Ophthalmology.* 2012;119:1066–1072

5. Michalewska Z, Michalewski J, Nawrocki J. Swept source optical coherence tomography of choroidal nevi. *Can J Ophthalmol.* 2016;51(4):271-276. doi: 10.1016/j.jcjo.2016.02.009.

6. Filloy A, Caminal JM, Arias L, Jordán S, Català J. Swept source optical coherence tomography imaging of a series of choroidal tumours. *Can J Ophthalmol.* 2015;50(3):242-248.

7. Singh AD, Mokashi AA, Bena JF, Jacques R, Rundle PA, Rennie IG. Small choroidal melanocytic lesions: Features predictive of growth. *Ophthalmology.* 2006;113(6):1032-1039.

8. Shields CL, Cater J, Shields JA, Singh AD, Santos MC, Carvalho C. Combination of clinical factors predictive of growth of small choroidal melanocytic tumors. *Arch Ophthalmol.* 2000;118(3):360-364.

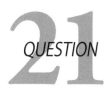

How Do I Distinguish One Pigmented Lesion From Another?

Amy C. Schefler, MD

Ryan S. Kim, BA

The differential diagnosis of a pigmented choroidal lesion includes choroidal nevus, choroidal melanoma, congenital hypertrophy of the retinal pigment epithelium (CHRPE), melanocytoma, extramacular disciform lesion, and other rarer entities. Given that a missed uveal melanoma diagnosis can be life-threatening, both general ophthalmologists and retinal specialists should be well versed in distinguishing these lesions from each other.

Choroidal Nevi and Melanoma

Pigmented choroidal nevi are extremely common in the White population, and it is estimated that 10% to 15% of adults have at least one such lesion. Uveal melanoma, on the other hand, is a rare disease with only 1200 to 2000 cases/year in the United States. Thus, the task of distinguishing a rare, but malignant lesion from many benign lesions is challenging. Funduscopic examination with fundus photography and ophthalmic ultrasound have long served as the core clinical diagnostic modalities in this endeavor. Gene expression profile (GEP) testing and multiplex ligand-dependent probe amplification, on the other hand, have become increasingly crucial in recent years for the management of uveal melanoma.[1,2]

While clinical findings via funduscopic exam and ultrasound are still an important part of monitoring choroidal lesions, both multiplex ligand-dependent probe amplification and GEP can help predict which melanoma patients will develop metastatic disease (Table 21-1). Thus, clinicians can use the genetic information to determine the prognosis and build a corresponding treatment regimen.

Fekrat S, ed. *Curbside Consultation in Retina: 49 Clinical Questions, Second Edition.* (pp 105-108).
© 2019 SLACK Incorporated

<table>
<tr><th colspan="3">Table 21-1
Gene Expression Profile Classifications
and Survival Data (Castle Biosciences)[3]</th></tr>
<tr><th>*Molecular Signature Class*</th><th>*Percent Metastasis Free at 3 Years*</th><th>*Percent Metastasis Free at 5 Years*</th></tr>
<tr><td>Class 1A</td><td>98%</td><td>98%</td></tr>
<tr><td>Class 1B</td><td>93%</td><td>79%</td></tr>
<tr><td>Class 2</td><td>50%</td><td>28%</td></tr>
</table>

Traditionally, various clinical features have been thought to be associated with growth of choroidal nevi into uveal melanoma, including orange pigmentation, presence of subretinal fluid and drusen, vascularity on B-scan ultrasonography, and low-to-medium internal reflectivity on A-scan ultrasonography. Recent data have also shown that increasing basal diameter confers additional poor prognosis in lesions with high-risk genomics.[4] Specifically, uveal melanoma that was classified as GEP Class 2 and had a basal diameter of less than 12 mm showed better prognosis than the larger counterpart.[5] Conversely, many of the clinicopathologic factors have recently been demonstrated not to exhibit a statistically significant association with GEP class and metastatic risk.[6]

Given that recent studies demonstrate that clinical features are not reliably predictive of the development and progression of uveal melanoma, performing a biopsy at the time of treatment for uveal melanoma has become an indispensable source of information for determining risk for metastasis. Genetic analysis may be extremely useful for confirming the diagnosis of melanoma and determining the prognosis. Moreover, based on the newer molecular data, the Class 1A genomic signature that is more common in smaller lesions will progress molecularly to Class 2 eventually in some cases. Therefore, clinicians are advised to treat patients as early as possible in order to minimize metastatic death.[7] It is best to consider both clinical features as well as genomic information for each melanoma.

Weighing all of the clinical risk factors associated with a particular lesion takes clinical experience and judgment. As a general rule, we feel that a patient with one or more high-risk features should be referred for assessment by an ocular oncologist (Figure 21-1). Small, flat, peripheral lesions (Figure 21-2) with no orange pigment and with associated drusen can be observed and documented with serial photography by a general ophthalmologist or retina specialist. When in doubt, an ophthalmologist who has limited experience with tumors should always refer a patient to an ocular oncologist for an evaluation.

Other Pigmented Choroidal Lesions

Other pigmented lesions that are important to include in the differential diagnosis of choroidal melanoma are CHRPE, melanocytoma, and extramacular disciform lesions associated with peripheral exudative hemorrhagic chorioretinopathy. These lesions are important to distinguish from choroidal nevi and melanoma. Distinguishing features are outlined in the following sections.

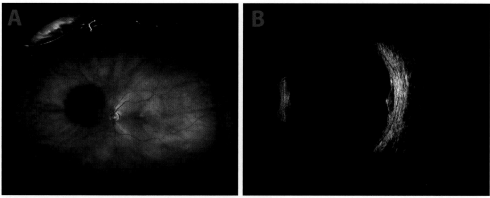

Figure 21-1. (A) A fundus photograph of a choroidal nevus is shown with high-risk characteristics, including apical thickness, orange pigment, and subretinal fluid. The 2 management options for this patient are close serial observation and plaque brachytherapy. (B) B-scan ultrasound image of the same eye demonstrating classic echographic hollowness.

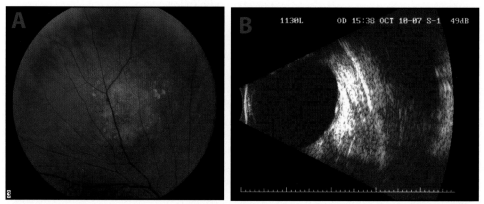

Figure 21-2. (A) Choroidal nevus is presented with low-risk characteristics, including no apical thickness, presence of drusen, no subretinal fluid, and lack of orange pigment. (B) B-scan ultrasound of the flat lesion in A is shown.

CONGENITAL HYPERTROPHY OF THE RETINAL PIGMENT EPITHELIUM

Its sharply demarcated borders and intralesional lacunae can distinguish CHRPE. They are generally flat, but the borders can enlarge slowly over time.[8] They can rarely occur within the macula, affecting central vision. When occurring as multiple lesions and configured in an oval shape, these lesions raise the suspicion for the diagnosis of Gardner syndrome, and such patients should be advised to undergo genetic testing and/or a colonoscopy to rule out cancerous polyps.

MELANOCYTOMA

Melanocytomas are typically jet black rather than the slate gray/brown hue of melanomas and most commonly occur in a peripapillary location (Figure 21-3) but can occur in the ciliary body or iris as well. They are much more common in Black patients than White patients. They most commonly demonstrate high internal reflectivity and avascularity on ultrasound. They can rarely have associated choroidal neovascularization or vascular occlusive events and can undergo small

Figure 21-3. This is a melanocytoma of the optic disc with typical jet-black pigment in a darkly pigmented individual.

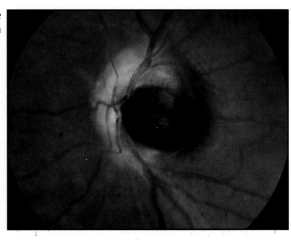

changes in size over time. There have been several rare reports of these lesions transforming into choroidal melanoma and as such, these lesions should be followed serially.

PERIPHERAL EXUDATIVE HEMORRHAGIC CHORIORETINOPATHY

An extramacular disciform lesion, also referred to as *peripheral exudative hemorrhagic chorioretinopathy*, can produce diagnostic confusion when associated with subretinal fluid, exudates, and/or vitreous hemorrhage. These can typically be distinguished from choroidal melanoma by their anterior location and presence of subretinal blood in various stages of resolution. While uveal melanomas can uncommonly be associated with subretinal hemorrhage, the degree of hemorrhage is not generally as profound as is its association with an extramacular disciform lesion. One helpful diagnostic clue is the presence of macular and/or peripheral drusen in association with the disciform lesion.

References

1. Onken MD, Worley LA, Tuscan MD, Harbour JW. An accurate, clinically feasible multi-gene expression assay for predicting metastasis in uveal melanoma. *J Mol Diagn.* 2010;12(4):461-468.
2. Schopper VJ, Correa ZM. Clinical application of genetic testing for posterior uveal melanoma. *Int J Retina Vitreous.* 2016;2:4.
3. Onken MD, Worley LA, Ehlers JP, Harbour JW. Gene expression profiling in uveal melanoma reveals two molecular classes and predicts metastatic death. *Cancer Res.* 2004;64(20):7205-7209.
4. Schefler A. Ocular Oncology Study Consortium (OOSC) report no 2: effect of clinical and pathologic variables on biopsy complication rates. Paper presented at: American Society of Retina Specialists. August 9-14, 2016; San Francisco, CA.
5. Walter SD, Chao DL, Feuer W, Schiffman J, Char DH, Harbour JW. Prognostic Implications of Tumor Diameter in Association With Gene Expression Profile for Uveal Melanoma. *JAMA Ophthalmol.* 2016;134(7):734-740.
6. Harbour JW. Association between choroidal nevus risk factors and gene expression profile prognostic class. Paper presented at: Retina Society. September 14-17, 2016; San Diego, CA.
7. Damato B. Progress in the management of patients with uveal melanoma. The 2012 Ashton Lecture. *Eye (Lond).* 2012;26(9):1157-1172.
8. Shields CL, Mashayekhi A, Ho T, Cater J, Shields JA. Solitary congenital hypertrophy of the retinal pigment epithelium: clinical features and frequency of enlargement in 330 patients. *Ophthalmology.* 2003;110(10):1968-1976.

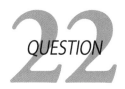

HOW DO I WORK UP AND MANAGE A PATIENT WITH A VITREOUS HEMORRHAGE?

Pauline T. Merrill, MD

Marina Gilca, MD

When evaluating a patient with a vitreous hemorrhage, the first step is to obtain a thorough history and perform a complete ophthalmic exam. On history, it is important to pay attention to specific ocular symptoms (eg, photopsias) or predisposing ocular conditions (eg, macular degeneration, myopia, retinal vein occlusion, macroaneurysm). The circumstances of vision loss may give additional clues (eg, trauma, valsalva). The past medical history may be notable for vascular systemic conditions, such as diabetes, hypertension, atherosclerosis, sickle cell anemia, or medications that could predispose to bleeding, including the newer oral anticoagulants (ie, rivaroxaban, apixaban, dabigatran). In children, there may be a history of retinopathy of prematurity, congenital/hereditary conditions associated with peripheral neovascularization (eg, Norrie disease, familial exudative vitreoretinopathy), or nonaccidental trauma.

On examination, visual acuity may correlate with the severity of the vitreous hemorrhage and/or the underlying pathology. The intraocular pressure may be low due to a retinal detachment or high due to neovascular glaucoma and may influence the timing of treatment. Important anterior segment findings include neovascularization of the iris or angle. Dilated ophthalmoscopic examination of both eyes allows you to evaluate the density of the hemorrhage as well as the underlying cause. If there is any view to the peripheral retina, look for retinal breaks or detachment with scleral depression. Areas of the fundus obscured by hemorrhage should be evaluated with B-scan ultrasonography. In addition to detecting a posterior vitreous detachment, flap tear, or retinal detachment, ultrasonography is also helpful in ruling out uncommon but important etiologies such as intraocular tumors. Fluorescein angiography may demonstrate abnormalities, such as neovascularization, ischemia, or macroaneurysm, not only in the fellow eye but also in eyes with mild or moderate vitreous hemorrhage.

Fekrat S, ed. *Curbside Consultation in Retina: 49 Clinical Questions, Second Edition.* (pp 109-111).
© 2019 SLACK Incorporated

Figure 23-1. FAF image of a healthy eye. Note the hypoautofluorescent disc and blood vessels as well as the hypoautofluorescent area in the fovea.

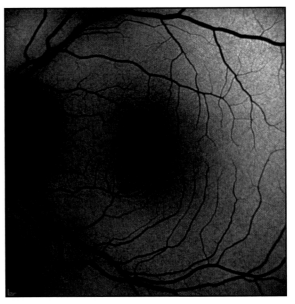

to facilitate interpretation and comparisons across patients and within the same patient over time. This approach is currently used to investigate different types of inherited, as well as acquired, macular diseases.

When 488-nm excitation is used in confocal scanning laser ophthalmoscopy modalities, such as Heidelberg Spectralis (Heidelberg Engineering), the normal FAF image shows a dark hypoautofluorescent disk and dark vessels and a grey to white isoautofluorescent background signal in the macula, except for the fovea. This is specific to 488-nm excitation wavelength where the normal macular pigment absorbs the excitation light, shielding the RPE from exposure to excitation and hence the hypoautofluorescence (Figure 23-1). This characteristic is not present when using green light FAF. Background FAF can vary widely between different patients, even in healthy eyes. Furthermore, FAF imaging itself causes a bleaching effect of the retinal photopigments, which appears as hyperautofluorescence of a previously imaged area. Hence, critical interpretation of FAF imaging is important and careful evaluation of colocalized SD-OCT imaging is advised in cases with ambiguous findings on FAF.

For the following retinal diseases, FAF has proven particularly useful: age-related macular degeneration (AMD), macular dystrophies, inherited retinal disorders, different types of drug toxicity, posterior uveitides, white dot syndromes, neoplastic and paraneoplastic retinal diseases as well as optic disc drusen.

For disorders involving the periphery of the ocular fundus, such as retinitis pigmentosa (RP), widefield imaging is recommended (especially as it uses green light) and is a great way to follow patients.

Age-Related Macular Degeneration

In AMD, FAF imaging is most helpful for evaluating the presence and extent of geographic atrophy (GA). GA is visualized as well-demarcated hypoautofluorescent areas surrounded by regions with varying degrees of hyperautofluorescence (Figure 23-2). Evaluation of foveal involvement is often challenging in patients with GA due to artifactual hypoautofluorescence caused by macular pigment (using 488 nm excitation). Therefore, we suggest ordering SD-OCT in all

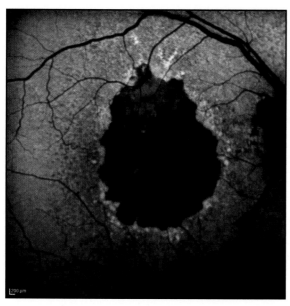

Figure 23-2. FAF image of the right eye of a patient with GA. The GA area is clearly demarcated as a hypoautofluorescent area, and has a well-defined hyperautofluorescent margin. Grainy hypoautofluorescence can be noted throughout the macula and even outside the arcades, consistent with reticular pseudodrusen.

patients with GA at baseline to unambiguously assess the condition of the fovea. FAF imaging, together with SD-OCT, is used as major outcome variable in randomized multicenter pharmaceutical trials evaluating the efficacy of novel drug treatment for GA. The presence of hyperautofluorescence at the border of GA has been used to characterize different types of GA patterns, of which some have significantly higher rates of progression (eg, diffuse trickling type).[5]

RPE rips may appear similar to GA, but often have dramatically angular shapes on FAF imaging. One way to distinguish the 2 entities on SD-OCT is the presence of elevated and folded RPE next to the area of RPE absence in the setting of RPE rips.

Drusen in AMD show variable degrees of autofluorescence depending on their type, size and the condition of the adjacent RPE, hence, we do not consider FAF particularly helpful in evaluating drusen.

Macular Dystrophies and Inherited Retinal Disorders

In Stargardt macular dystrophy, FAF typically shows a central hypoautofluorescent lesion corresponding to RPE atrophy surrounded by multiple bright, hyperautofluorescent flecks in the posterior pole.[6] In patients with late onset or slowly progressive variants, the FAF picture can aid in differentiating this entity from advanced AMD, which may present a similar clinical picture. Pattern dystrophies, a heterogenous group of maculopathies caused by mutations in the peripherin/retinal degeneration slow gene, are characterized by abnormalities in FAF. Adult-onset vitelliform dystrophy, for example, may resemble AMD clinically and by OCT; however, it can often be distinguished from AMD by the presence of very symmetrical and bilateral accumulations of hyperautofluorescent material in the fovea.

In RP, a group of hereditary generalized photoreceptor dystrophies, widefield FAF is a helpful imaging modality for early detection of peripheral changes, which may be missed clinically. Patchy hypoautofluorescent areas in the periphery may be an early finding in RP and should prompt the clinician to order electroretinography testing or genetic testing to confirm the diagnosis. Furthermore, the presence of a hyperautofluorescent ring around the fovea, delineating the transition from normal to abnormal photoreceptors, is one of the hallmarks of RP. In contrast to

Figure 23-3. FAF image of the right eye of a patient demonstrating chloroquine toxicity. A well-demarcated grainy hypoautofluorescent ring around the fovea can be noted indicating photoreceptor and RPE damage, surrounded by a ring of hyperautofluorescence, indicating early photoreceptor changes.

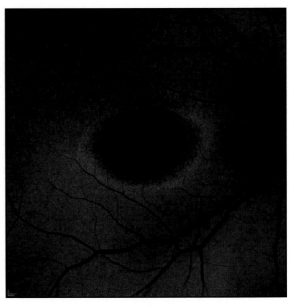

cone and cone/rod dystrophies, where a hyperautofluorescent ring can be found as well, the ring in RP patients constricts over time, whereas a longitudinal enlargement of the ring can be observed in patients with cone or cone/rod dystrophy.[7]

Drug Toxicity

In patients currently or previously treated with chloroquine or hydroxychloroquine, FAF is a valuable adjunct to the primary screening tests (SD-OCT plus automated visual fields), because it provides a topographic view of retinal and RPE damage secondary to drug toxicity. FAF shows early photoreceptor damage as hyperautofluorescent areas, typically located parafoveally, with later changes involving RPE atrophy appearing hypoautofluorescent (Figure 23-3).[8] This is of particular value in Asian patients who have been shown to frequently develop more peripheral paramacular lesions (along the arcades) in Plaquenil (hydroxychloroquine) toxicity, which could be missed when using SD-OCT or the usual 10-2 visual fields.[9] Therefore, we suggest that FAF imaging be incorporated in patients with a history of Plaquenil treatment, as an adjunct to SD-OCT.

Didanosine, a nucleoside reverse transcriptase inhibitor, previously used for treatment of HIV, can cause retinal toxicity, leading to peripheral retinal atrophy resembling the clinical appearance of choroideremia in advanced stages. Widefield FAF imaging therefore has clinical value in screening for drug toxicity and documenting longitudinal changes of RPE pathology.[10]

Posterior Uveitis and White Dot Syndromes

In several posterior uveitides, such as serpiginous choroiditis, active lesions are characterized by hyperautofluorescence, whereas old, healed lesions are hypoautofluorescent. FAF is helpful in monitoring and detecting active vs old and inactive lesions. Similarly, in multifocal choroiditis, active lesions are hyperautofluorescent, whereas old atrophic lesions are hypoautofluorescent. In addition, FAF may detect large zones of photoreceptor disruption around these focal inflammatory lesions, which may otherwise be missed on OCT.[11]

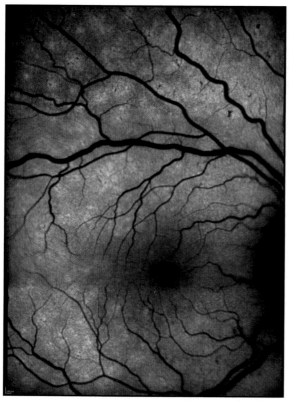

Figure 23-4. FAF montage image of the right eye of a patient with multiple evanescent white dot syndrome. Hyperautofluorescent areas, which are partially confluent, correspond to white spots seen clinically and correspond to outer photoreceptor loss, unmasking the normal RPE autofluorescence.

In acute zonal occult outer retinopathy (AZOOR), FAF shows the trizonal sign, consisting of isoautofluorescence outside the AZOOR lesion, patchy hyperautofluorescence in subacute lesions and hypoautofluorescence within old lesion areas, corresponding to RPE atrophy.[12] Furthermore, in some cases of AZOOR, a transient yellowish demarcation line can be observed, surrounding the AZOOR lesion. This line has been shown to be best appreciated by FAF imaging.[12]

In multiple evanescent white dot syndrome, FAF typically shows hyperautofluorescent areas corresponding to the white dots seen clinically (Figure 23-4).

Neoplastic and Paraneoplastic Diseases

In cases of intraocular lymphoma, which may resemble drusen on SD-OCT imaging, FAF can often help make the diagnosis by revealing bright hyperautofluorescent spots, which help distinguish lymphoma from AMD.

Autoimmune retinopathy shows hyperautofluorescence co-localized with loss of outer retinal structures on SD-OCT. A hyperautofluorescent ring surrounding an area of normal FAF in the macula may be found.

Optic Disc Drusen

In cases where a clear distinction between papilledema and optic disc drusen cannot be made clinically, FAF can provide great value. Optic disc drusen, especially when superficially located in the disc structure, usually show bright hyperautofluorescence, which can easily differentiate them from optic disc swelling secondary to other causes.

Summary

FAF is a fast and noninvasive imaging method, which is a valuable adjunct *en face* imaging modality in a variety of retinal diseases. We find that in certain conditions, FAF can add complimentary and often diagnostic clues to standard imaging modalities, such as SD-OCT.

References

1. Delori FC, Dorey CK, Staurenghi G, Arend O, Goger DG, Weiter JJ. In vivo fluorescence of the ocular fundus exhibits retinal pigment epithelium lipofuscin characteristics. *Invest Ophthalmol Vis Sci.* 1995;36(3):718-729.
2. Yung M, Klufas MA, Sarraf D. Clinical applications of fundus autofluorescence in retinal disease. *Int J Retina Vitreous.* 2016;2:12.
3. Keilhauer CN, Delori FC. Near-infrared autofluorescence imaging of the fundus: visualization of ocular melanin. *Invest Ophthalmol Vis Sci.* 2006;47(8):3556-3564.
4. Heiferman MJ, Fawzi AA. Discordance between blue-light autofluorescence and near-infrared autofluorescence in age-related macular degeneration. *Retina.* 2016;36(Suppl 1):S137-S146.
5. Holz FG, Bindewald-Wittich A, Fleckenstein M, et al. Progression of geographic atrophy and impact of fundus autofluorescence patterns in age-related macular degeneration. *Am J Ophthalmol.* 2007;143(3):463-472.
6. Cukras CA, Wong WT, Caruso R, Cunningham D, Zein W, Sieving PA. Centrifugal expansion of fundus autofluorescence patterns in Stargardt disease over time. *Arch Ophthalmol.* 2012;130(2):171-179.
7. Oishi A, Oishi M, Ogino K, Morooka S, Yoshimura N. Wide-field fundus autofluorescence for retinitis pigmentosa and cone/cone-rod dystrophy. *Adv Exp Med Biol.* 2016;854:307-313.
8. Marmor MF, Kellner U, Lai TY, Melles RB, Mieler WF; American Academy of Ophthalmology. Recommendations on screening for chloroquine and hydroxychloroquine retinopathy (2016 revision). *Ophthalmology.* 2016;123(6):1386-1394.
9. Melles RB, Marmor MF. Pericentral retinopathy and racial differences in hydroxychloroquine toxicity. *Ophthalmology.* 2015;122(1):110-6.
10. Haug SJ, Wong RW, Day S, et al. Didanosine retinal toxicity. *Retina.* 2016;36(Suppl 1):S159-S167.
11. Munk MR, Jung JJ, Biggee K, et al. Idiopathic multifocal choroiditis/punctate inner choroidopathy with acute photoreceptor loss or dysfunction out of proportion to clinically visible lesions. *Retina.* 2015;35(2):334-343.
12. Mrejen S, Khan S, Gallego-Pinazo R, Jampol LM, Yannuzzi LA. Acute zonal occult outer retinopathy: a classification based on multimodal imaging. *JAMA Ophthalmol.* 2014;132(9):1089-1098.

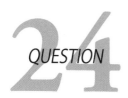

WHAT ADDITIONAL INFORMATION CAN I GET FROM ULTRA-WIDEFIELD FLUORESCEIN ANGIOGRAPHY THAT I CAN'T GET FROM A 30-DEGREE ANGIOGRAM?

Jeremy A. Lavine, MD, PhD
Justis P. Ehlers, MD

Standard 7-field 30° fluorescein angiography (FA) is the historical gold standard for the diagnosis and monitoring of many retinal diseases. In focal macular diseases, such as pseudophakic cystoid macular edema, age-related macular degeneration, myopic degeneration, and other causes of posterior pole choroidal neovascularization, 30° angiography with or without sweeps will often determine the diagnosis. However, there are several retinal diseases, including inflammatory eye disease, retinal vascular disease, and peripheral retinal lesions, that may be more optimally assessed with ultra-widefield fluorescein angiography (UWFFA), which images 200° of retina.

Retinal Vascular Diseases

Diabetic retinopathy and retinal venous occlusive disease are the 2 most common retinal vascular disorders. UWFFA may facilitate diagnosis, disease burden assessment, and help guide management. In diabetic retinopathy, macular leakage, macular ischemia, and posterior neovascularization may be detected on standard 7-field 30° FA with sweeps. In Figure 24-1A, neovascularization of the disc is evident, the superior nasal sweep identifies retinal neovascularization elsewhere, and the inferior sweeps show blockage from vitreous hemorrhage (blue asterisk). However, a single focal area of ischemia is only visualized on the nasal sweep (red asterisk). Instead, with UWFFA, the massive ischemic burden in the temporal periphery is identified (green asterisk). Equipped with this information, panretinal laser photocoagulation can be performed with a priority to the areas of peripheral nonperfusion. In Figure 24-1B, the standard 7-field 30° FA demonstrates no

Fekrat S, ed. *Curbside Consultation in Retina: 49 Clinical
Questions, Second Edition.* (pp 119-124).
© 2019 SLACK Incorporated

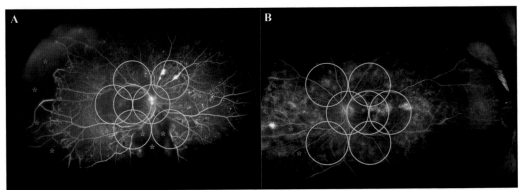

Figure 24-1. Comparative assessment of simulated standard angiography and UWFFA in diabetic retinopathy. (A) On simulated 7-field imaging, neovascularization of the disc is evident and the superior nasal sweep identifies posterior neovascularization (magenta asterisk) and the inferior sweeps show blockage from vitreous hemorrhage (blue asterisk). A focal area of ischemia is noted inferonasally on a single sweep (red asterisk). With UWFFA, massive ischemic burden in the temporal periphery is now identified (green asterisk). (B) Simulated 7-field angiography identifies diffuse leakage, but UWFFA impacts the diagnosis due to nasal neovascularization (magenta asterisk) and ischemia (green asterisk).

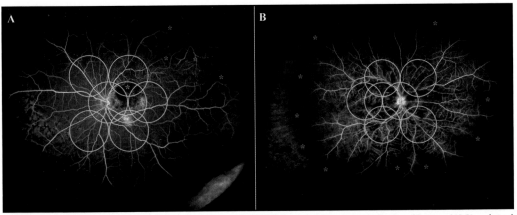

Figure 24-2. Simulated standard angiography and UWFFA in retinal venous occlusive disease. (A) Simulated 7-field imaging for a BRVO that exhibits blockage from hemorrhage (blue asterisk) in the macula. No clear ischemia is detected. UWFFA identifies significant nonperfusion (green asterisk) and vascular remodeling (magenta asterisk). (B) Imaging for a central retinal vein occlusion with blockage from hemorrhage in all standard 7-field 30° sweeps and limited visualization of ischemia (red asterisk). UWFFA illustrates massive ischemia (green asterisk) and nonperfusion in all of 4 quadrants of the periphery.

significant ischemia or neovascularization; however, the UWFFA displays nasal neovascularization (magenta asterisk) and ischemia (green asterisk). Overall, UWFFA in diabetic retinopathy is particularly useful for localizing ischemia, determining extent of ischemia, identifying peripheral neovascularization, and assessing overall disease burden.

Retinal vein occlusions may be diagnosed with standard 30° angiography, but the evaluation of disease burden is significantly limited compared to UWFFA. In Figure 24-2A, a branch retinal vein occlusion (BRVO) is shown with blockage from hemorrhage (blue asterisk) in the macula and superior temporal periphery. In the standard 7-field 30° FA, no ischemia is detectable, and this BRVO would be classified as non-ischemic according to the Branch Vein Occlusion Study.[1] However, with UWFFA, the superotemporal periphery demonstrates extensive nonperfusion (green asterisk) and vascular remodeling (magenta asterisk), consistent with significant ischemia.

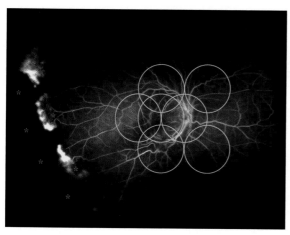

Figure 24-3. Sickle cell retinopathy. Simulated 7-field angiography demonstrates vascular tortuosity, whereas UWFFA illustrates massive temporal ischemia (green asterisk) and sea fan neovascularization (magenta asterisk).

Figure 24-2B demonstrates a central retinal vein occlusion with blockage from hemorrhage in all standard 7-field 30° sweeps and only focal ischemia in the temporal sweep (red asterisk) and thus, might be considered non-ischemic.[2] Conversely, the UWFFA illustrates massive ischemia (green asterisk) and nonperfusion in all of 4 quadrants of the periphery. In this case example, enhanced surveillance and close follow-up will be encouraged to evaluate for neovascularization given the extensive ischemia identified on UWFFA.

Beyond diabetic retinopathy and retinal vein occlusions, UWFFA can be invaluable for the diagnosis and management of other retinal vascular diseases, including ocular ischemic syndrome and hemoglobinopathies, especially sickle cell trait and sickle cell disease. In Figure 24-3, the standard 30° fields appear normal; however, the UWFFA illustrates massive temporal ischemia (green asterisk) and sea fan neovascularization (magenta asterisk), confirming the diagnosis of proliferative sickle cell retinopathy.

Uveitis

The utility of FA is well described for the diagnosis of specific uveitic entities. However, the usefulness of UWFFA for the diagnosis and management of inflammatory eye disease is becoming more apparent. UWFFA of intermediate uveitis with petaloid macular leakage (blue asterisk), disc leakage (red asterisk), and peripheral vascular leakage (green asterisk) is shown in Figure 24-4A. After treatment with oral steroids, standard 7-field FA demonstrates persistent petaloid macular leakage (blue asterisk) and leakage of the optic nerve head (red asterisk) in Figure 24-4B. The amount of petaloid macular and disc leakage appears roughly stable compared to before steroid therapy. However, UWFFA imaging illustrates clear improvement in the peripheral vascular leakage (magenta asterisk), which would have been missed on standard 30° angiography.

Identification of overall leakage burden in uveitis can also be facilitated with UWFFA. In another example of intermediate uveitis, no macular or disc leakage is shown (Figure 24-5A). The central area of blockage is due to a posterior subcapsular cataract (blue asterisk). The peripheral sweeps identify a small to moderate amount of peripheral leakage, but the UWFFA allows for visualization of far greater leakage in the periphery (green asterisk). After steroid therapy, evaluation of overall treatment response and reduction in peripheral vascular leakage (magenta asterisk) is more completely enabled with UWFFA.

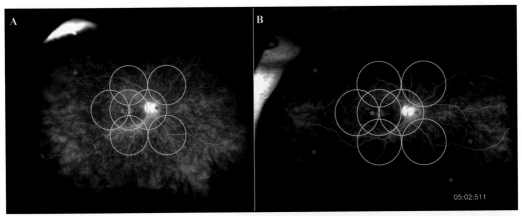

Figure 24-4. Angiography options in uveitis. (A) Extensive leakage identified on simulated 7-field FA with petaloid macular leakage (blue asterisk) and disc leakage (red asterisk). Ultra-widefield angiography also confirms peripheral vascular leakage (green asterisk). (B) Following treatment, 7-field FA demonstrates persistent but slightly improved macular leakage (blue asterisk) and leakage of the optic nerve head (red asterisk) but does provide information on improvement of extensive peripheral vascular leakage (magenta asterisk).

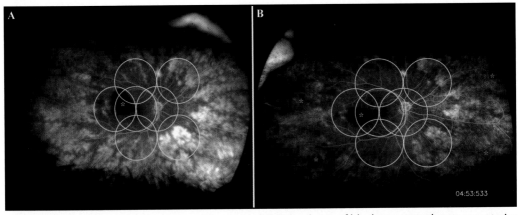

Figure 24-5. Leakage burden assessment in uveitis. (A) Central area of blockage secondary to a posterior subcapsular cataract (blue asterisk). The peripheral sweeps identify a small-moderate amount of leakage, while ultra-widefield imaging reveals extensive additional leakage. (B) Following therapy, significant improvement is particularly visualized with ultra-widefield angiography (magenta asterisk).

The utility of UWFFA for the management of intermediate and posterior uveitis has been evaluated.[3] In this study, ultra-widefield imaging changed management decisions in 33% of patients compared to standard 30° imaging. In addition to intermediate uveitis, UWFFA may be particularly useful in retinal vasculitis, masquerade syndromes, diagnostic dilemmas, infectious uveitis, and Susac syndrome.

Peripheral Retinal Lesions

Standard 7-field imaging is limited in capturing far peripheral lesions. UWFFA provides a unique opportunity to provide imaging of entire peripheral retinal lesions. Peripheral exudative hemorrhagic chorioretinopathy (PEHCR) typically presents as a peripheral elevated lesion that

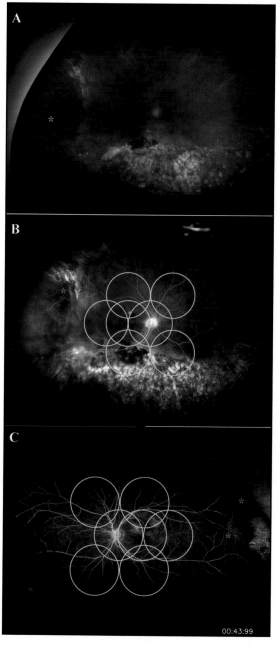

Figure 24-6. Peripheral lesions and ultra-widefield imaging. (A) Color photo demonstrates peripheral dark mass lesion with associated hemorrhage (blue asterisk). (B) Minimal view of peripheral lesion is noted with simulated 7-field imaging. Macular leakage from possible choroidal neovascularization (red asterisk) is identified. Ultra-widefield imaging confirms blockage from hemorrhage (green asterisk) and associated leakage (magenta asterisk), facilitating diagnosis of PEHCR. (C) In a separate example, ultra-widefield angiography demonstrating extensive temporal peripheral nonperfusion (green asterisk) with vascular remodeling and light bulb-type aneurysmal changes (magenta asterisk), whereas the simulated 7-field 30° FA demonstrated only macular vascular remodeling.

may simulate malignant choroidal melanoma.[4] Comprehensive imaging of these lesions can help facilitate diagnosis. In PEHCR, ultra-widefield imaging demonstrates a large temporal subretinal lesion (blue asterisk), poorly focused macula with hemorrhage, and inferior retinal pigment epithelial changes with hemorrhage (Figure 24-6A). The UWFFA (Figure 24-6B) shows blockage from hemorrhage and macular leakage from a choroidal neovascular membrane (red asterisk) in the simulated 7-field 30° angiogram. The ultra-widefield image demonstrates the temporal subretinal lesion with blockage from hemorrhage (green asterisk) and leakage from the choroidal neovascularization superior to the lesion (magenta asterisk). No intrinsic vasculature or other features consistent with choroidal melanoma are detected. The ultra-widefield area also reveals the widespread inferior retinal pigment epithelial changes (blue asterisk) consistent with PEHCR.

In addition to PEHCR and choroidal melanoma, UWFFA is useful for the diagnosis of vaso-proliferative tumors, intraocular lymphoma, multifocal central serous chorioretinopathy, Coat disease, and other peripheral retinal tumors and retinal lesions. UWFFA can expand the differential diagnosis. In one example, simulated 7-field 30° FA shows macular vascular remodeling (red asterisk) with leakage in the superior macula (Figure 24-6C). However, UWFFA identifies extensive temporal peripheral nonperfusion (green asterisk) with vascular remodeling and light bulb-type aneurysmal changes (magenta asterisk), suggesting a potential diagnosis of Type I macular telangiectasia or possibly atypical Coat disease.

Summary

Standard 7-field 30° FA provides important information regarding macular disease assessment. However, UWFFA is a new standard for panretinal assessment of retinal disease and may be particularly useful for retinal vascular disease, inflammatory eye disease, masquerade syndromes, diagnostic dilemmas, and peripheral retinal lesions. UWFFA demonstrates excellent utility in the identification of peripheral retinal ischemia, documentation of disease burden, and detection of disease activity/peripheral vascular leakage. Additional research is needed for the development of quantitative metrics and pattern-based assessments to fully utilize the extensive information contained in UWFFA.

References

1. Branch Vein Occlusion Study Group. Argon laser scatter photocoagulation for prevention of neovascularization and vitreous hemorrhage in branch vein occlusion. A randomized clinical trial. *Arch Ophthalmol.* 1986;104:34-41.
2. Central Vein Occlusion Study Group. A Randomized clinical trial of early panretinal photocoagulation for ischemic central vein occlusion. The Central Vein Occlusion Study Group N report. *Ophthalmology.* 1995;102:1434-1444.
3. Campbell JP, Leder HA, Sepah YJ, et al. Wide-field Retinal Imaging in the Management of Noninfectious Posterior Uveitis. *Am J Ophthalmol.* 2012;154:908-911.e2.
4. Shields CL, Salazar PF, Mashayekhi A, Shields JA. Peripheral exudative hemorrhagic chorioretinopathy simulating choroidal melanoma in 173 eyes. *Ophthalmology.* 2009;116:529-535.

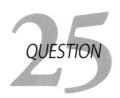

WHAT IMAGING OPTIONS ARE THERE TO DETECT AN INTRAOCULAR FOREIGN BODY? WHEN DO I GET WHICH ONE?

Daniel G. Cherfan, MD
Sumit Sharma, MD

Open globes, regardless of the mechanism of injury, can result in significant loss of vision and may often result in multiple surgeries with poor outcomes depending on the extent of damage. Open globe injuries (OGI) can be further complicated by the presence of an intraocular foreign body (IOFB) in 18% to 41% of cases of penetrating ocular trauma.[1] The detection of an IOFB is crucial in determining the management plan and surgical approach to globe repair, although this can be difficult at times due to a limited view into the affected eye. Imaging is almost always indicated and should not be delayed for penetrating globe injuries when there is any suspicion of an IOFB.

History and Examination

Detection of an IOFB starts with an extensive history of the incident and a complete clinical examination. A detailed description of the mechanism of injury in the setting of an open globe can help determine whether one or more IOFBs should be suspected. Having an idea of the general timing of an injury can also influence the next appropriate step in management. Determining the composition and characteristics of the IOFB can dictate what imaging studies are ordered and the overall management of the patient.

A thorough examination at the slit-lamp is crucial in any case of a suspected OGI with the possibility of an IOFB. Other than direct visualization of an IOFB, clinical signs such as small self-sealing wounds, iris transillumination defects, corectopia, sectoral cataract, vitreous hemorrhage,

Fekrat S, ed. *Curbside Consultation in Retina: 49 Clinical Questions, Second Edition.* (pp 125-130).
© 2019 SLACK Incorporated

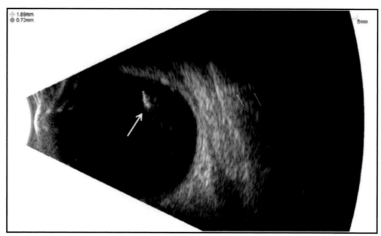

Figure 25-2. Hyperreflectivity of IOFB (white arrow) on B-scan with linear reverberation echos (comet tail sign; colored arrows).

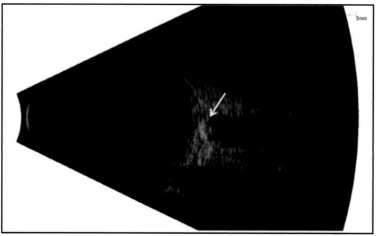

Figure 25-3. B-scan of patient with suspected IOFB. Evidence of an IOFB located in Tenon space with marked shadowing (white arrow).

Additionally, ultrasound biomicroscopy (UBM) is particularly helpful in the case of known or occult anterior segment IOFBs. The high frequency of UBM provides a detailed view of anterior structures and their relation to an IOFB which can be very helpful in determining the surgical approach. IOFBs located within the angle, embedded in the ciliary body, or in the posterior chamber may go undetected on clinical exam and are not easily identified on conventional imaging. In these cases, anterior segment imaging with UBM allows for the identification of such occult IOFBs (Figure 25-5).

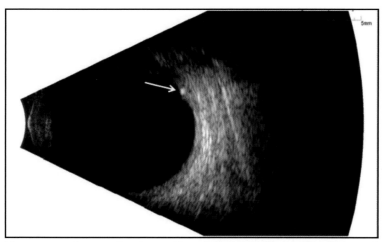

Figure 25-4. B-scan of patient with an IOFB embedded within the retinal tissue (white arrow).

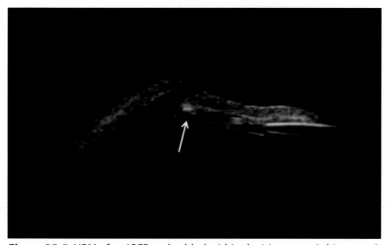

Figure 25-5. UBM of an IOFB embedded within the iris stroma (white arrow).

What to Do Next

Presence of an IOFB poses a significantly higher risk of developing endophthalmitis and thus intravenous antibiotics should be administered immediately. Vancomycin (1 g every 12 hours) and ceftazidime (1 g every 12 hours) are excellent choices in order to provide broad-spectrum coverage against both Gram-positive and Gram-negative organisms that commonly cause endophthalmitis in the setting of an IOFB. The patient may need a tetanus shot. Surgical removal of the IOFB is always almost indicated and should ideally be done at the time of the open globe repair in order to minimize the risk of developing endophthalmitis or retinal detachment. We usually inject intra-vitreal broad-spectrum antibiotics following removal of acute IOFBs. If a vitreoretinal surgeon is not available to assist with removal of an IOFB, then primary closure of the OGI should be performed to minimize the risk of developing endophthalmitis and the patient should be referred to an experienced surgeon for removal of the IOFB as soon as possible.

References

1. Loporchio D, Mukkamala L, Gorukanti K, et al. Intraocular foreign bodies: a review. *Surv Ophthalmol*. 2016;61:582-596.
2. Allon G, Beiran I, Seider N, Blumenthal EZ. The role of computed tomography in the immediate workup of open globe injury. *Eur J Ophthalmol*. 2016;26:503-4.
3. Liu CC, Tong JM, Li PS, Li KK. Epidemiology and clinical outcome of intraocular foreign bodies in Hong Kong: a 13-year review. *Int Ophthalmol*. 2017;37:55-61.
4. Pinto A, Brunese L, Daniele S, et al. Role of computed tomography in the assessment of intraorbital foreign bodies. *Semin Ultrasound CT MR*. 2012;33:392-395.
5. Zhang Y, Cheng J, Bai J, et al. Tiny ferromagnetic intraocular foreign bodies detected by magnetic resonance imaging: a report of two cases. *J Magn Reson Imaging*. 2009;29:704-707.

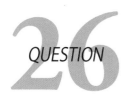

WHY WOULD I WANT TO LOOK AT CHOROIDAL THICKNESS ON OPTICAL COHERENCE TOMOGRAPHY?

Glenn Yiu, MD, PhD

The practice of measuring choroidal thickness became prevalent with the advent of enhanced depth imaging optical coherence tomography (EDI-OCT). First described by Spaide et al,[1] EDI-OCT is a specialized mode of OCT that takes advantage of the greater depth attained from the inverted image one gets by placing the OCT device closer to the subject's eye. Today, many current generation spectral domain OCT systems have a software mode that automates this process and produces an OCT image that provides much higher quality cross-sectional visualization of the choroidal vasculature as well as the choroid-scleral junction. By measuring the distance between Bruch membrane and the choroid-scleral junction at various locations in the macula, it became possible to measure choroidal thickness across a spectrum of retinal and choroidal diseases (Figure 26-1).

Before we discuss which conditions are best distinguished by looking at choroidal thickness, it is important to note that, unlike measuring the thickness of the retina, which consists of neural tissue, the choroid is a vascular structure that can vary significantly between individuals. Choroidal thickness decreases linearly with age, undergoing 20 to 30 mm of thinning with each decade of adult life.[2] The thickness of the choroid is also strongly associated with axial length and refractive error with highly myopic eyes having the thinnest choroid. Finally, choroidal thickness also varies with time of day, being thicker in the morning and thinnest in the evening, such that measurements taken at different times on consecutive visits may not be easily compared with each other. Hence, while the general rule of thumb is that normal choroidal thickness is roughly equal to the thickness of the retina in the central macula, it is important to take into account the patient's age, refractive error, and the time of day at which the OCT image was taken. To add to the complexity, the posterior boundary of the choroid (ie, the choroid-scleral junction) is not

Fekrat S, ed. *Curbside Consultation in Retina: 49 Clinical Questions, Second Edition.* (pp 131-135).
© 2019 SLACK Incorporated

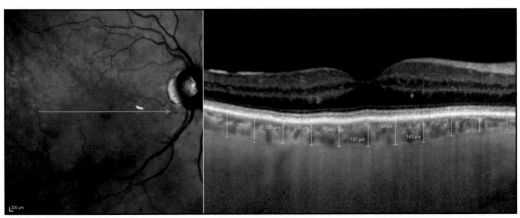

Figure 26-1. Choroidal thickness measurements on EDI-OCT. Infrared and EDI-OCT image of a cross-section of the macula of a normal eye, showing caliper measurements of choroidal thickness at the fovea and at 500 μm intervals nasal and temporal to the fovea. Measurements are taken from Bruch membrane to the choroid-scleral junction at the posterior border of the choroid stroma. The green arrow on the infrared image corresponds to the location of the EDI-OCT image.

always clearly delineated, with a portion of normal individuals demonstrating a visible suprachoroidal space between the choroid stroma and sclera.[3] Hence, there is still significant controversy on how the choroid should be precisely measured and hardly any commercially available software can reproducibly segment the choroid or automatically generate a choroidal thickness measurement. So, at the current time, most eyecare providers must rely on manual choroidal segmentation or manual measurements of choroidal thickness using calipers integrated into the OCT software.

With these considerations in mind, I think the most useful clinical application for measuring choroidal thickness is in diagnosing retinal conditions that are classified as a pachychoroid spectrum condition, such as central serous chorioretinopathy (CSC). The term *pachychoroid*, derived from the Greek term *pachy* meaning thick, refers to a collection of related retinal disorders that are characterized by abnormal thickening and dilation of choroidal vessels and increased choroidal hyperpermeability. Examples include CSC and polypoidal choroidal vasculopathy (PCV), and the nomenclature has expanded to include pachychoroid pigment epitheliopathy, which refers to changes that are considered precursors to CSC, and pachychoroid neovasculopathy, which describes Type I choroidal neovascularization in eyes with pachychoroid pigment epitheliopathy or CSC.[4] I find that obtaining EDI-OCT is particularly useful in eyes with subretinal fluid and vascular leakage on fluorescein angiography that may resemble exudative age-related macular degeneration (AMD), but may also result from chronic CSC or atypical PCV. Even in an elderly patient with drusen and pigment changes, there is significant overlap between these conditions in clinical and angiographic appearance. Especially in cases where subretinal fluid responds poorly to repeated anti-vascular endothelial growth factor (anti-VEGF) therapy, I would consider obtaining EDI-OCT to evaluate the choroidal vasculature. The presence of a thick choroid (Figure 26-2), particularly in the presence of large choroidal vessel lumen, would support a diagnosis of PCV or CSC and potentially benefit from photodynamic therapy, or in the case of CSC, the use of oral mineralocorticoid antagonists, such as eplerenone. Using additional imaging modalities to characterize the choroid, such as indocyanine green angiography or novel OCT angiography (OCT-A), could further clarify the etiology of the condition. Interestingly, recent studies have also shown that the choroid becomes thinner with successful photodynamic therapy treatment of CSC and PCV, suggesting that tracking choroidal thickness changes may be a means of monitoring treatment response.

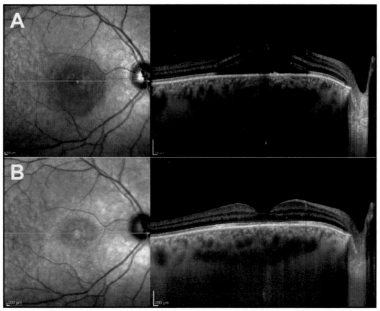

Figure 26-2. Thickened choroid in CSC. (A) Infrared and EDI-OCT images showing subretinal macular fluid and thickened choroid in an eye with CSC at the time of diagnosis, and (B) resolution of fluid after observation for 4 months without intervention. The green arrow on the infrared images corresponds to the location of the EDI-OCT images.

Another useful application of EDI-OCT is for distinguishing choroidal lesions or tumors that may be too small to be characterized on B-scan ultrasonography.[5] Amelanotic nevi appear homogenous with medium reflectivity and visible choroidal vessels, while melanotic nevi and choroidal melanomas appear highly reflective in the anterior choroid with shadowing and poor visualization of the choroidal vessels. Choroidal hemangiomas have medium-to-low reflectivity without shadowing, while choroidal metastases have low reflectivity in the deep choroid with enlargement of the suprachoroidal space. Comparisons between EDI-OCT and ultrasonography have shown that OCT is more accurate and reproducible for measuring the lesion height, especially when using systems where image registration allows measuring the lesion at the same location between visits. In contrast, B-scans tend to overestimate actual tumor size. EDI-OCT is also extremely useful for distinguishing choroidal lesions from scleral lesions, such as sclerochoroidal calcifications, where the choroid is distinctly compressed from the underlying scleral protrusions (Figure 26-3).

The applications of choroidal thickness measurements continue to expand as we learn more about the pathophysiology of more common retinal diseases, such as AMD or diabetic macular edema, although the actual clinical utility in these conditions remain unclear at the current time. The choroid appears thinner in patients with AMD, but this correlation may be confounded by the fact that AMD worsens with age, so it becomes difficult to distinguish natural age-related choroidal thinning from pathologic changes. Nevertheless, several lines of evidence have shown that eyes with reticular pseudodrusen and geographic atrophy are associated with choroidal thinning, which may even predict visual outcomes.[6] Similarly, the choroid has been found to be thinner in eyes with diabetic macular edema, but some of this effect may in part result from anti-VEGF therapy.[7] As VEGF is an important growth factor that is involved in the physiologic maintenance of the choroidal vasculature, it seems reasonable that chronic VEGF antagonism could result in adverse secondary effects on the health of the choroid. In these cases, rapid thinning of the choroid in the setting of many repeated anti-VEGF injections may portend the onset of geographic atrophy.

Figure 26-3. Choroidal imaging of sclerochoroidal calcifications. (A) Fundus photo, (B) infrared, and (C) EDI-OCT image of an eye with sclerochoroidal calcifications. Notice that the choroid is not thickened, but the underlying sclera is protruding from below. There are small areas of subretinal fluid at the apex of the more prominent lesion. The highlighted green line on the infrared image corresponds to the location of the EDI-OCT image.

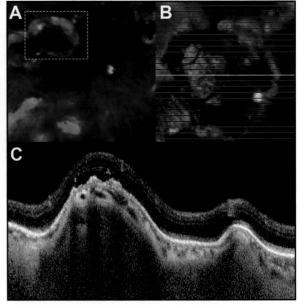

Choroidal thickness has also been evaluated across a spectrum of uveitic conditions. In particular, Vogt-Koyanagi-Harada syndrome, which often presents with a phenotype similar to CSC, has been associated with choroidal thickening. Successful treatment of Vogt-Koyanagi-Harada with steroids is also accompanied by a reduction in choroidal thickness, again suggesting the potential of using choroidal thickness as a parameter to monitor response to treatment. The choroid may also be thicker in posterior scleritis and posterior uveitides, such as Behcet disease, or thinner in cases of birdshot chorioretionpathy. While many studies have shown that choroidal thickness may be affected in various conditions, it is important to again note that choroidal thickness is highly variable and difficult to measure reliably on OCT, with reproducibility studies showing a minimum of at least 40 to 50 mm difference to distinguish true clinical change from measurement variability.[8] Thus, with the recent explosion of published work in this area, it is important to pay careful attention when interpreting the literature.

Summary

Evaluating choroidal thickness on OCT can be incredibly helpful, particularly when used to distinguish pachychoroid spectrum disorders from AMD or for diagnosing certain types of choroidal lesions or tumors. Newer swept source OCT systems employ longer wavelength light sources that allow even better visualization of deeper structures within the choroid. With the advent of OCT-A and other *en face* methods of visualizing choroidal structure, clinicians must pay attention not only to the overall thickness of the choroid, but also to anatomic structures within the choroidal layers, such as the presence of thickened vessels, polyps, or neovascularization.

References

1. Spaide RF, Koizumi H, Pozzoni MC. Enhanced depth imaging spectral-domain optical coherence tomography. *Am J Ophthalmol*. 2008;146(4):496-500.
2. Abbey AM, Kuriyan AE, Modi YS, et al. Optical coherence tomography measurements of choroidal thickness in healthy eyes: correlation with age and axial length. *Ophthalmic Surg Lasers Imaging Retina*. 2015;46(1):18-24.
3. Yiu G, Pecen P, Sarin N, et al. Characterization of the choroid-scleral junction and suprachoroidal layer in healthy individuals on enhanced-depth imaging optical coherence tomography. *JAMA Ophthalmol*. 2014;132(2):174-181.
4. Dansingani KK, Balaratnasingam C, Naysan J, Freund KB. En face imaging of pachychoroid spectrum disorders with swept-source optical coherence tomography. *Retina*. 2016;36(3):499-516.
5. Torres VL, Brugnoni N, Kaiser PK, Singh AD. Optical coherence tomography enhanced depth imaging of choroidal tumors. *Am J Ophthalmol*. 2011;151(4):586-593, e582.
6. Kang HM, Kwon HJ, Yi JH, Lee CS, Lee SC. Subfoveal choroidal thickness as a potential predictor of visual outcome and treatment response after intravitreal ranibizumab injections for typical exudative age-related macular degeneration. *Am J Ophthalmol*. 2014;157(5):1013-1021.
7. Yiu G, Manjunath V, Chiu SJ, Farsiu S, Mahmoud TH. Effect of anti-vascular endothelial growth factor therapy on choroidal thickness in diabetic macular edema. *Am J Ophthalmol*. 2014;158(4):745-751, e742.
8. Vuong VS, Moisseiev E, Cunefare D, Farsiu S, Moshiri A, Yiu G. Repeatability of choroidal thickness measurements on enhanced depth imaging optical coherence tomography using different posterior boundaries. *Am J Ophthalmol*. 2016;169:104-112.

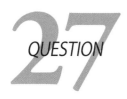

WHEN SHOULD I REFER A PATIENT WITH AN EPIRETINAL MEMBRANE AND WHAT IF THERE IS ASSOCIATED CYSTOID MACULAR EDEMA?

Gaurav K. Shah, MD
Daniel Connors, MD

An epiretinal membrane (ERM) is a disorder of the vitreomacular interface resulting in tangential tractional force on the retina leading to macular thickening and distortion. There is great variation in presentation with some patients visually asymptomatic and others with significant morbidity, including metamorphopsia and reduced vision. Pathologically, it is a result of fibrocellular proliferation on the innermost surface of the retina.[1,2]

The prevalence of ERM varies based on the population being studied, with rates ranging from 2.2% to 18.5%, the incidence increasing with age.[3] An ERM may be classified as primary or idiopathic, or secondary. A variety of common ocular conditions are known to be associated with ERM formation including diabetic retinopathy, retinal vein occlusion, history of retinal break or detachment, or trauma. While the exact cause of an idiopathic ERM is inherently unclear, it is believed to be due to anomalous posterior vitreous detachment.[1] Anomalous posterior vitreous detachment is the result of vitreous liquefaction occurring faster than the weakening of vitreoretinal adhesion, resulting in tractional forces on the retina. This traction is proinflammatory and causes the release of a variety of cytokines resulting in fibrocellular proliferation[1] (Figure 27-1). When evaluating a patient with an ERM, it is important to keep the etiologies of a secondary ERM in mind. Patients should specifically be evaluated for the presence of retinal vascular disease, uveitis, or an occult retinal break.

ERMs are often asymptomatic in the early stages, and the majority of these membranes remain stable after an initial period of growth. Progression, however, may lead to significant visual impairment, metamorphopsia, macropsia, diplopia, and even aniseikonia. It is especially important to ask these patients about symptoms of visual distortion that can occur in the setting of

Fekrat S, ed. *Curbside Consultation in Retina: 49 Clinical Questions, Second Edition.* (pp 137-140).
© 2019 SLACK Incorporated

Figure 27-1. ERM with premacular fibrosis.

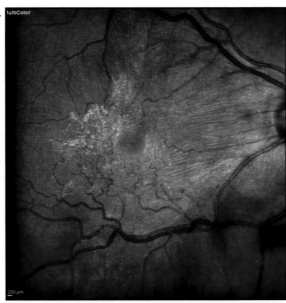

Figure 27-2. ERM with retinal thickening on OCT.

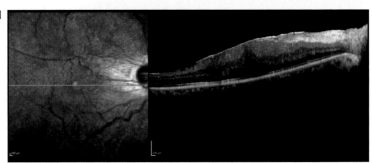

normal visual acuity. In many cases, Snellen visual acuity may not be consistent with the patient's symptomatic complaints, and this may be more evident in those with professions that demand high visual quality (eg, pilots, physicians, nurses, engineers).

Optical coherence tomography (OCT) is a noninvasive imaging technique that produces a cross-sectional view of the retina and is now the primary method of imaging ERMs (Figure 27-2). OCT has proven to be more sensitive in identifying an ERM than clinical examination and has largely supplanted fluorescein angiography. Images are obtained using light to produce extremely high-resolution images from within biological tissues.

Often, an ERM may be identified in a patient with nonspecific visual complaints. It falls on the clinician to determine if the membrane is significant and whether it warrants referral to a retina specialist for evaluation. As the incidence of ERM and cataract both increase with age, it is not uncommon for patients to present with both a visually significant cataract as well as an ERM. The patient with a significant ERM will complain more of distorted vision than decreased vision. He or she will note straight lines appear wavy and that images are larger or smaller in the eye with the membrane than in the unaffected eye. As surgical intervention to remove the ERM results in cataract progression typically within the first year, cataract surgery prior to vitrectomy is indicated in patients with significant lens changes.

Reassurance, an Amsler grid for home monitoring, and periodic follow-up are sufficient for a patient with an idiopathic ERM and minimal visual symptoms. If the patient is troubled by the visual symptoms caused by the ERM, or a causative process, such as retinal vascular disease or retinal tear is noted, referral to a vitreoretinal surgeon is the next step. In the past, surgery was usually reserved for 2 categories of patients: (1) visual acuity of 20/60 or less, or (2) those patients that required excellent visual acuity or a high degree of stereopsis. Improvements in surgical technique and intraoperative ERM visualization as well as reduced complication rates now allow for earlier vitrectomy and removal of the ERM irrespective of presenting acuity. A series of patients treated at The Retina Institute for ERM with 20/40 vision or better had improved visual outcomes following surgery.[3]

A thin membrane, short duration of symptoms, and the absence of traction are all factors leading to a better postoperative prognosis.[2,4] In one meta-analysis evaluating 411 eyes with idiopathic ERM, 70% demonstrated stable or improved visual acuity with 40% to 50% improving by more than 2 lines after ERM peeling.[5] Another study that specifically examined quality of life following surgery found a dramatic improvement in metamorphopsia following surgery.[6]

Patients that undergo removal of the ERM should be aware that complications of surgery may include increased intraocular pressure, hemorrhage, retinal detachment, and especially cataract progression. Recurrence of the ERM has been previously reported to occur in approximately 10% of patients. More recently, however, Schadlu and colleagues[4] found that when the internal limiting membrane was removed in conjunction with peeling of the ERM, there was recurrence in only 1/38 patients at the 20-month follow-up.

What If There Is Associated Cystoid Macular Edema?

Cystoid macular edema (CME) as a result of tractional forces exerted on the retina can contribute to reduced visual acuity and metamorphopsia in patients with an ERM. Fluid accumulates in the outer plexiform and inner nuclear layers of the retina in a cystic pattern. Fluorescein angiography will demonstrate early hyperfluorescence consistent with leakage in a petaloid pattern as dye accumulates in the cystic spaces. This will also be readily apparent on OCT. Identifying the cause of the edema is essential in determining its treatment. While CME as a result of a vein occlusion, diabetes, or macular degeneration can result in rapid visual loss, tractional edema typically does not progress rapidly and doesn't necessarily require urgent treatment. While topical steroids and non-steroidal anti-inflammatory agents can be utilized in the treatment of CME secondary to an ERM, pars plana vitrectomy with membrane peel is frequently indicated. Given recent advances in surgical technique, smaller gauge surgery, and improving outcomes, surgical intervention provides a very high chance for success.

References

1. Stevenson W, Prospero Ponce CM, Agarwal DR, Gelman R, Christoforidis JB. Epiretinal membrane: optical coherence tomography-based diagnosis and classification. *Clin Ophthalmol.* 2016;10:527-534.
2. Almony A, Nudleman E, Shah GK, et al. Techniques, rationale, and outcomes of internal limiting membrane peeling. *Retina.* 2012;32(5):877-891.
3. Chinskey N, Fine H, Shah G. Practical update to epiretinal membrane. *OSLI Retina.* 2016;47(7):614-616
4. Schadlu R, Tehrani S, Shah GK, Prasad AG. Long-term follow-up results of ILM peeling during vitrectomy surgery for premacular fibrosis. *Retina.* 2008;28(6):853-857.
5. Roh M, Kim EL, Eliott D, Yonekawa Y. Internal limiting membrane peeling during idiopathic epiretinal membrane removal: pros and cons. *J Vitreoretin Dis.* 2017;1(2):138-143.
6. Ghazi-Nouri SMS, Tranos PG, Rubin GS, Adams ZC, Charteris DG. Visual function and quality of life following vitrectomy and epiretinal membrane peel surgery. *Br J Ophthalmol.* 2006;90(5):559-562.

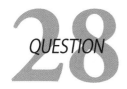

How Do I Differentiate A Macular Hole From A Lamellar Hole From An Epiretinal Membrane With A Pseudohole, And Why Do I Care?

SriniVas R. Sadda, MD

Optical coherence tomography (OCT) has proven to be a critical tool in the evaluation of the vitreoretinal interface.[1] In addition to providing high-resolution cross-sectional images of the neurosensory retina, OCT is also capable of demonstrating the relationship between the posterior hyaloid and the retina—a relationship that is difficult to assess by clinical examination alone. In fact, when OCT imaging was first introduced in the early 1990s, the ability to distinguish similar yet distinct conditions, such as macular hole, lamellar hole, epiretinal membrane (ERM) with pseudohole, and vitreomacular traction (VMT) syndrome, was among the first really useful clinical applications of the new technology. Further advances in OCT, including the development of high-speed, highly-sensitive swept source OCT technology has allowed the vitreoretinal relationships to be understood in even greater detail (Figure 28-1), and for the steps in the evolution of vitreous detachment to be identified.

Prior to the introduction of OCT, there were many hypotheses, but only limited evidence regarding the pathogenesis of macular hole and associated disorders. While there is still more to be learned, it is now clear that macular hole, ERM, and related vitreomacular interface (VMI) disorders are due to abnormalities in the normal vitreous separation process.[2] The normal process of vitreous detachment involves progressive liquefaction of the vitreous (leading to increased mobility) as well as weakening of the adhesion between the vitreous and retina. Defects in this normal process can lead to these VMI diseases. For example, if liquefaction of the vitreous gel outpaces the weakening of the adhesion, vitreous movements can lead to traction on the retina at points of continued attachment (eg, at the fovea).[2] This traction results in structural changes at the foveal center and ultimately the formation of a macular hole or related condition. Alternatively,

Fekrat S, ed. *Curbside Consultation in Retina: 49 Clinical
Questions, Second Edition.* (pp 141-147).
© 2018 SLACK Incorporated

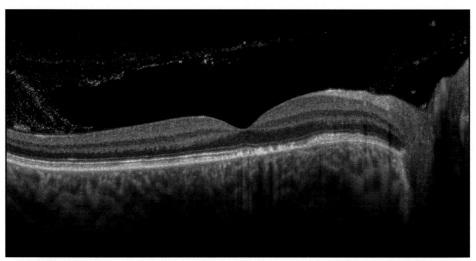

Figure 28-1. Swept source OCT B-scan of the optic disc and macula. Note the high level of detail where the vitreous, and its attachments at the optic nerve and temporal to the macula, can be seen. Areas of liquefaction or vitreoschisis are also readily apparent overlying the macula.

in some cases, the main body of the cortical vitreous separates, but small bits of residual vitreous remain adherent to the retinal surface. These residual islands of vitreous may form the nidus for subsequent epiretinal proliferation.

This improved understanding of the pathophysiology of these vitreoretinal disorders and the broad availability of OCT allowed the development of a new international consensus classification of VMI diseases.[2] This new classification system also identifies specific features to define and differentiate these disorders and includes specific subclassifications that help define the appropriate management.

Full-Thickness Macular Holes

Full-thickness macular hole (FTMH) formation is age-related, typically occurring in postmenopausal women. A staging system for macular holes was originally suggested by Johnson and Gass[3] and subsequently adapted (with minor modifications). In these original staging systems, a Stage I hole was defined by pseudocyst formation in the inner retina (Figure 28-2), which sometimes may be seen clinically as a yellow dot or ring. This was thought to be an important stage to recognize clinically, since in many cases, spontaneous resolution was possible. In Stage II, there is early separation of the outer photoreceptor layer and, consequently, small full-thickness loss of retinal tissue (Figure 28-3). Stage III occurs when the hole is greater than 400 μm in diameter with surrounding thickened retina, including intraretinal cystoid spaces. Stage IV holes consist of Stage III holes with a complete posterior vitreous detachment (Figure 28-4). Although not originally defined by Johnson and Gass, some investigators also defined a Stage 0 hole to refer to the fellow eye with vitreomacular adhesion (VMA) (but no traction) of a patient with FTMH in the one eye—such an eye was thought to still be at risk for developing a FTMH. Prior to the advent of OCT, the subjective disappearance of a portion of a slit beam of light (Watzke-Allen test) or a laser aiming beam projected into the hole was a useful method for distinguishing a FTMH from other vitreoretinal interface disorders. Despite its widespread use, this staging system had several obvious limitations. For example, patients with small holes (eg, < 400 μm) could develop vitreous separation (see Figure 28-4). Such a hole would then be considered a Stage IV hole though it may

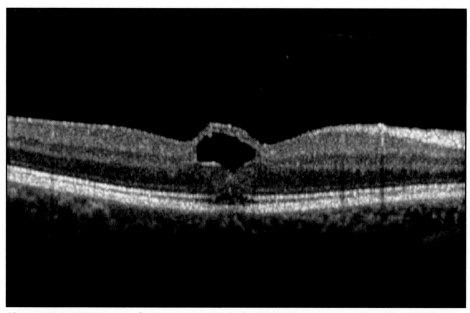

Figure 28-2. OCT B-scan of a Stage I macular hole. Note the inner retinal cyst, but the absence of a full-thickness retinal defect. In the new classification system, this would be termed *vitreomacular traction.*

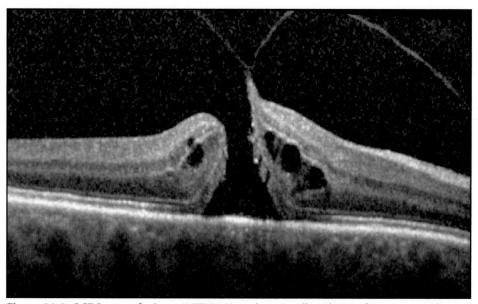

Figure 28-3. OCT B-scan of a Stage II FTMH. Note there is still evidence of vitreous attachment, and the width of the hole at the level of the external limiting membrane measures less than 250 µm. In the new classification system, this would be termed a *small macular hole with VMT.*

be smaller than a larger Stage III hole with some persistent vitreous attachment. Due to these inconsistencies, and to provide a classification system that would be relevant to pharmacologic and surgical therapeutics, the International Vitreomacular Traction Study (IVTS) group was convened.[2] The IVTS system classified holes based on size and presence or absence of traction.

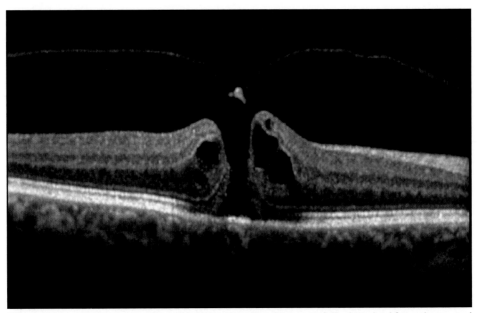

Figure 28-4. OCT B-scan of a Stage IV FTMH. Note the vitreous is fully detached from the central macula and an opacity can be seen in the overlying detached hyaloid. This opacity is often termed a *pseudo-operculum*. In the new classification system, this would be termed a *small macular hole without VMT*.

The old term Stage 0 hole was replaced by VMA. The term Stage I hole or impending macular hole was replaced by VMT. VMA and VMT were distinguished based on demonstrable morphological changes in the retina in the setting of VMT (see Figure 28-2). FTMH were classified as having VMT present or absent and also classified by size as small (aperture < 250 µm), medium (250 to 400 µm), and large (> 400 µm). The cutoff of 250 µm for small holes was based on the fact that these holes do have a small rate of spontaneuous closure, a very high closure rate with vitrectomy,[4,5] and the most favorable outcome with pharmacologic vitreolysis (eg, ocriplasmin).[6,7] The cutoff of 400 µm was chosen because these holes were unlikely to close with pharmacologic approaches. This new system does not easily align with the old Gass system. A Gass Stage II hole would be a small or medium FTMH with VMT with the new system (see Figure 28-3). A Gass Stage III hole would be a medium or large FTMH with VMT, and a Gass Stage IV hole would be small (see Figure 28-4), medium, or large FTMH without VMT. Regardless, the recognition of FTMH hole is of critical importance as it defines an eye that likely will need therapeutic intervention.

Lamellar Holes

The term *lamellar hole* was first suggested by Donald Gass as a complication of chronic cystoid macular edema following cataract extraction. It is now more commonly thought to represent an aborted process in the spectrum of macular hole formation (ie, a lamellar hole occurs when VMT causes unroofing of a foveal pseudocyst without loss of the outer photoreceptor layer).[8,9] The IVTS group identified several features of a lamellar macular hole (LMH) including: (1) irregular foveal contour, (2) defect in the inner retina, (3) intraretinal schisis, and (4) intact photoreceptors at the base (ie, not an FTMH) (Figure 28-5). Most patients with this condition complain of mild symptoms of metamorphopsia and may have only limited central vision loss. On biomicroscopy, these

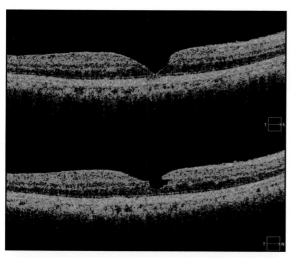

Figure 28-5. Two OCT B-scans of an eye with a LMH. Note irregular contour of the retina and thinning of the outer nuclear layer. This thinning of the outer retina allows this lesion to be distinguished from an ERM with pseudohole. Absence of a full-thickness defect of the retina distinguishes this from a FTMH.

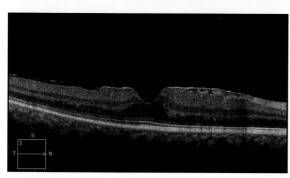

Figure 28-6. OCT B-scan of an eye with an ERM and early pseudohole. Note steepening of the foveal pit due to dragging or traction from the ERM, which appears as a thin hyperreflective structure on the retinal surface. Unlike a lamellar hole, there is no thinning of the outer retina.

lesions appear as round or oval reddish lesions. These lesions tend to progress slowly and many remain stable. They may expand or progress more rapidly, however, in the presence of adjacent vitreopapillary traction. Surgery for these lesions remains controversial, and prospective studies are needed.[10-12]

Epiretinal Membrane and Pseudoholes

Centripetal contraction of an ERM can lead to formation of a distinct clinical entity, the pseudohole.[1,13,14] Pseudoholes may have a similar clinical appearance to a FTMH or a lamellar hole and may appear as a circular red spot on biomicroscopy. The key difference is that there is no loss of foveal tissue in pseudoholes.[15] OCT characteristics of a pseudohole include steepened foveal pit with thickened edges, reduced foveal pit diameter, normal or slightly increased foveal thickness, and concomitant ERM (Figure 28-6). Even with the use of OCT, it may be difficult to distinguish between a pseudohole and a lamellar hole in some cases because severe dragging on the inner retina by the ERM may make the fovea appear thinned. Sometimes the dragging can be sufficiently severe that an overhang is observed. Like lamellar holes, pseudoholes tend to be relatively stable conditions, and the visual acuity of affected patients may be relatively preserved.[13] Cystoid macular edema, significant metamorphopsia, or vision loss associated with the ERM may precipitate surgical intervention.[16]

Why Do I Care?

It is important to differentiate macular holes from lamellar holes and pseudoholes because the management is different in each case. Vitrectomy surgery and gas tamponade are well-established and successful treatment options for FTMH.[4,5,17] More recently, for smaller holes with focal VMT, Jetrea (ocriplasmin) may be an option.[6,7] ERM peeling may be beneficial for the treatment of visually significant pseudoholes. On the other hand, treatment of patients with significant visual loss from a lamellar hole remains controversial, with many reports noting adverse outcomes, such as progression to FTMH formation. Although successful outcomes after vitrectomy have also been reported in such cases,[10] caution is still required.

References

1. Mirza RG, Johnson MW, Jampol LM. Optical coherence tomography use in evaluation of the vitreoretinal interface: a review. *Surv Ophthalmol*. 2007;52(4):397-421. doi: 10.1016/j.survophthal.2007.04.007
2. Duker JS, Kaiser PK, Binder S, et al. The International Vitreomacular Traction Study Group classification of vitreomacular adhesion, traction, and macular hole. *Ophthalmology*. 2013;120(12):2611-9. doi: 10.1016/j.ophtha.2013.07.042.
3. Johnson RN, Gass JD. Idiopathic macular holes. Observations, stages of formation, and implications for surgical intervention. *Ophthalmology*. 1988;95(7):917-24.
4. Ben Simon GJ, Desatnik H, Alhalel A, Treister G, Moisseiev J. Retrospective analysis of vitrectomy with and without internal limiting membrane peeling for stage 3 and 4 macular hole. *Ophthalmic Surg Lasers Imaging*. 2004;35(2):109-15.
5. Ezra E, Gregor ZJ; Morfields Macular Hole Study Group Report N. Surgery for idiopathic full-thickness macular hole: two-year results of a randomized clinical trial comparing natural history, vitrectomy, and vitrectomy plus autologous serum: Morfields Macular Hole Study Group Report no. 1. *Arch Ophthalmol*. 2004;122(2):224-36. doi: 10.1001/archopht.122.2.224
6. Dugel PU, Tolentino M, Feiner L, Kozma P, Leroy A. Results of the 2-Year Ocriplasmin for Treatment for Symptomatic Vitreomacular Adhesion Including Macular Hole (OASIS) randomized trial. *Ophthalmology*. 2016;123(10):2232-47. doi: 10.1016/j.ophtha.2016.06.043
7. Stalmans P, Benz MS, Gandorfer A, et al. Enzymatic vitreolysis with ocriplasmin for vitreomacular traction and macular holes. *N Engl J Med*. 2012;367(7):606-15. doi: 10.1056/NEJMoa1110823
8. Michalewska Z, Michalewski J, Odrobina D, Nawrocki J. Non-full-thickness macular holes reassessed with spectral domain optical coherence tomography. *Retina*. 2012;32(5):922-9. doi: 10.1097/IAE.0b013e318227a9ef
9. Witkin AJ, Ko TH, Fujimoto JG, et al. Redefining lamellar holes and the vitreomacular interface: an ultrahigh-resolution optical coherence tomography study. *Ophthalmology*. 2006;113(3):388-97. doi: 10.1016/j.ophtha.2005.10.047.
10. Garretson BR, Pollack JS, Ruby AJ, Drenser KA, Williams GA, Sarrafizadeh R. Vitrectomy for a symptomatic lamellar macular hole. *Ophthalmology*. 2008;115(5):884-6, e1. doi: 10.1016/j.ophtha.2007.06.029
11. Sato T, Emi K, Bando H, Ikeda T. Retrospective comparisons of vitrectomy with and without air tamponade to repair lamellar macular hole. *Ophthalmic Surg Lasers Imaging Retina*. 2015;46(1):38-43. doi: 10.3928/23258160-20150101-06
12. Spaide RF. Closure of an outer lamellar macular hole by vitrectomy: hypothesis for one mechanism of macular hole formation. *Retina*. 2000;20(6):587-90.
13. Byon IS, Pak GY, Kwon HJ, Kim KH, Park SW, Lee JE. Natural history of idiopathic epiretinal membrane in eyes with good vision assessed by spectral-domain optical coherence tomography. *Ophthalmologica*. 2015;234(2):91-100. doi: 10.1159/000437058

14. Liu X, Ling Y, Huang J, Zheng X. Optic coherence tomography of idiopathic macular epiretinal membranes. *Yan Ke Xue Bao*. 2002;18(1):14-9.
15. Michalewski J, Michalewska Z, Dziegielewski K, Nawrocki J. Evolution from macular pseudohole to lamellar macular hole-spectral domain OCT study. *Graefes Arch Clin Exp Ophthalmol*. 2011;249(2):175-8. doi: 10.1007/s00417-010-1463-1.
16. Miliatos I, Lindgren G. Epiretinal membrane surgery evaluated by subjective outcome. *Acta Ophthalmol*. 2017;95(1):52-9. doi: 10.1111/aos.13001
17. Parravano M, Giansanti F, Eandi CM, Yap YC, Rizzo S, Virgili G. Vitrectomy for idiopathic macular hole. *Cochrane Database Syst Rev*. 2015;(5):CD009080. doi: 10.1002/14651858.CD009080.pub2

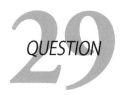
WHAT IS MICROPULSE LASER
AND WHAT CAN IT BE USED FOR?

Scott D. Walter, MD, MSc

Although anti-vascular endothelial growth factor (anti-VEGF) therapy has become the mainstay of treatment for many retinovascular diseases, laser therapy remains an important therapeutic option for many patients. In fact, more than 45% of patients enrolled in Protocol T received laser photocoagulation (focal, grid, or both) due to persistent diabetic macular edema (DME) despite 6 or more months of rigorous anti-VEGF therapy[1]; whereas conventional focal or grid laser treatments involve retinal photocoagulation and resultant scar formation, newer treatment paradigms, such as micropulse laser (IRIDEX Corporation) and subthreshold continuous wave laser are intended to achieve therapeutic photostimulation of the retinal pigment epithelium (RPE) without photocoagulation of the overlying neurosensory retina. While we are still learning about the optimal indications and treatment parameters for this technology, I use micropulse laser as adjunctive therapy in a majority of my patients with persistent center-involving DME despite anti-VEGF therapy, and as primary therapy in select patients with macular edema from various causes.

Multiple factors contribute to the development of macular edema, including increased vascular permeability, an inflammatory milieu, and RPE pump dysfunction or exhaustion. Because macular edema is such a multifactorial disease, the use of multiple treatment modalities targeting different aspects of the disease pathophysiology may be required in order to achieve an optimal treatment response. Whereas anti-VEGF and steroid injections primarily target vascular permeability and inflammatory pathways respectively, the target of micropulse laser is the RPE.

Pigmented RPE cells absorb more laser energy than transparent retinal elements due to differences in their absorption spectra. Conventional laser photocoagulation works by heating the RPE and overlying photoreceptors to greater than 60°C, resulting in coagulative necrosis of ischemic retina, in turn reducing VEGF production. The postulated mechanism of action for micropulse

Fekrat S, ed. *Curbside Consultation in Retina: 49 Clinical
Questions, Second Edition.* (pp 149-152).
© 2019 SLACK Incorporated

laser is completely different. *In vitro* experiments suggest that therapeutic laser-tissue interactions may occur at lower, sublethal levels of RPE thermal stimulation: RPE cells upregulate heat shock proteins and other cellular rejuvenation pathways, essentially triggering tissue-healing responses without killing any RPE cells or overlying photoreceptors. This sublethal RPE stimulation is hypothesized to enhance the RPE's ability to pump intraretinal fluid out of the retina, across the outer blood-retinal barrier, and into the choroidal outflow tract.

Conventional laser photocoagulation results in retinal whitening during the procedure and subsequent chorioretinal scar formation in the following weeks to months; however, when micropulse laser is performed correctly, there should be no visible changes to the retina during or after laser treatment. When applying irradiances less than 350 W/cm^2, there are no detectable signs of laser-induced retinal injury even by infrared, red-free, fundus autofluorescence, or optical coherence tomography imaging.[2] In fact, micropulse laser can be directly applied to the fovea without causing treatment-associated vision loss or evidence of structural damage to the retina on multimodal imaging.[3] For those accustomed to visible laser burns, micropulse laser may seem almost homeopathic due to the lack of a visible endpoint. For me, adopting this technology required a leap of faith and some patience to wait and see the treatment effects materialize. Efficacy can be assessed by monitoring reduction of macular thickness observed 1 to 2 months following treatment.

Subvisible laser-tissue interactions are achieved with the micropulse setting by modifying duty cycle. With continuous wave laser, the duty cycle is automatically set to 100%, and the laser emission is constant throughout the pulse duration. A 50% duty cycle means that the instrument delivers a series of interrupted (50% on/50% off) pulses; and a 5% duty cycles means that the instrument delivers a series of 5% on/95% off pulses. With a shorter duty cycle, a shorter pulse width limits the spread of laser-induced tissue hyperthermia, and a longer interval between pulses allows time for tissue cooling before the next pulse is delivered. MicroPulse Laser Therapy (IRIDEX) thereby allows selective thermal stimulation of the RPE in a finely controlled fashion.

I have experience performing micropulse laser with a frequency-doubled 577 nm neodymium-doped yttrium-aluminum-garnet laser (Fovea-Friendly MicroPulse Laser Therapy platform by IRIDEX) using a 5 % duty cycle and a pulse duration of 200 ms (Figure 29-1A). In the micropulse mode, there is a built-in repetition rate of 500 Hz, such that the duration of each micropulse is only 0.1 ms with a 1.9 ms rest between pulses (Figure 29-1B); therefore, each 200 microseconds (ms) laser emission consists of 100 micropulses totaling 10 ms on and 190 ms off (Figure 29-1C). The Arrhenius integral is a measure of tissue injury calibrated such that 1.0 equals the limit of cellular viability. With conventional laser photocoagulation, the Arrhenius integral exceeds 1.0, resulting in cellular coagulation and necrosis. However, the Arrhenius integral is approximately 10-fold lower with micropulse laser and subthreshold continuous wave laser; moreover, the energy uptake is more selectively targeted towards the RPE with micropulse laser (Figure 29-1D).

Micropulse capabilities are also available on an 810 nm diode laser platform (IRIDEX OcuLight SLx). A recent randomized controlled trial suggests similar safety and efficacy with either yellow (577 nm) or infrared (810 nm) wavelength micropulse laser.[4] Subthreshold continuous wave laser treatment can be achieved by systematically reducing the laser energy by 70% after determining the threshold for a barely visible burn (PASCAL EndPoint Management System by Topcon). Whether any substantive differences exist between these 2 approaches to subthreshold laser is not yet established in the literature.

Micropulse laser has demonstrated efficacy for DME,[2-5] macular edema from retinal vein occlusion,[2] and central serous retinopathy (CSR).[6] Many patients with these conditions demonstrate an incomplete response to anti-VEGF therapy, and I will often add micropulse laser as an adjunct to anti-VEGF treatment rather than switching anti-VEGF agents or resorting to steroids. In patients with center-involving DME, I routinely recommend micropulse laser to those who respond poorly or incompletely after 3 to 6 doses of anti-VEGF therapy. Not all patients respond

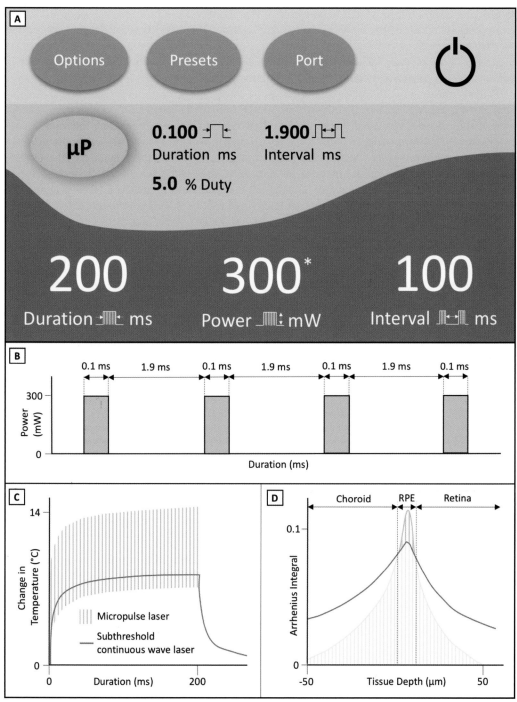

Figure 29-1. (A) My standard settings for 577 nm micropulse laser. Note (*) that power is adjusted between 300 and 400 mW depending on the degree of fundus pigmentation. (B) A train of 4 micropulse cycles illustrating micropulse width, amplitude, and interval with these settings. (C) Conceptual model of tissue warming and (D) injury with 200 ms emission of subthreshold laser using 500 Hz micropulse (orange) vs continuous wave laser (red). Note that micropulse laser generates a series of 100 temperature spikes and cooling periods, whereas continuous wave laser generates a lower but sustained elevation of tissue temperature over 200 ms. At equivalent pulse duration and energy, micropulse laser concentrates more energy on the target tissue (RPE) and causes less tissue injury to adjacent structures (choroid and retina).

to a single session, but most will demonstrate a significant reduction in macular edema if 2 or 3 treatments are performed over the span of several months. It is important to educate patients that the therapeutic response to micropulse laser is less immediate but often more durable than other treatment options. In my experience, micropulse laser can help to reduce injection frequency in patients treated concurrently with anti-VEGF therapy.

Primary treatment with micropulse laser can be considered in the appropriate clinical circumstances. While I would normally initiate anti-VEGF as first-line therapy in patients with macular edema from diabetes or retinal vein occlusion, I am comfortable recommending micropulse laser as primary therapy in patients with 20/20 visual acuity and those who are reluctant to begin injections for other reasons. Micropulse laser is quick to perform and generally well-tolerated, making it an ideal first line therapy for patients with heightened procedural anxiety. A recent meta-analysis concluded that superior visual acuity outcomes were achieved in treatment-naïve patients with DME treated with micropulse laser vs conventional laser photocoagulation.[5] Keep in mind that micropulse laser will not photocoagulate microaneurysms, and the treatment may need to be combined with conventional focal laser in order to address both components of the disease. I also like to offer micropulse laser as primary therapy in CSR. A small randomized controlled trial with an observational arm suggested that micropulse laser had efficacy similar to photodynamic therapy for CSR.[6] Typically, I wait 3 to 6 months before considering photodynamic or pharmacologic therapy for central serous, but there is little harm in trying micropulse laser in the meantime with the aim of stimulating subretinal fluid reabsorption by the RPE.

References

1. Wells JA, Glassman AR, Ayala AR, et al; Diabetic Retinopathy Clinical Research Network. Aflibercept, bevacizumab, or ranibizumab for diabetic macular edema. *N Engl J Med.* 2015; 372:1193-1203.
2. Luttrull JK, Sramek C, Palanker D, Spink CJ, Musch DC. Long-term safety, high-resolution imaging, and tissue temperature modeling of subvisible diode micropulse photocoagulation for retinovascular macular edema. *Retina.* 2012; 32:375-386.
3. Luttrull JK, Sinclair SH. Safety of transfoveal subthreshold diode micropulse laser for fovea-involving diabetic macular edema in eyes with good visual acuity. *Retina.* 2014; 34:2010-2020.
4. Vujosevic S, Martini F, Longhin E, Convento E, Cavarzeran F, Midena E. Subthreshold micropulse yellow laser versus subthreshold micropulse infrared laser in center-involving diabetic macular edema. *Retina.* 2015; 35:1594-1603.
5. Chen G, Tzekov R, Li W, Jiang F, Mao S, Tong Y. Subthreshold micropulse diode laser versus conventional laser photocoagulation for diabetic macular edema: a meta-analysis of randomized controlled trials. *Retina.* 2016; 36:2059-2065.
6. Kretz FT, Beger I, Koch F, Nowomiejska K, Auffarth GU, Koss MJ. Randomized clinical trial to compare micropulse photocoagulation versus half-dose verteporfin photodynamic therapy in the treatment of central serous chorioretinopathy. *Ophthalmic Surg Lasers Imaging Retina.* 2015;46:837-843.

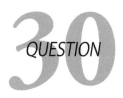

WHAT IS THE TREATMENT PARADIGM FOR POSTOPERATIVE PSEUDOPHAKIC MACULAR EDEMA?

Felipe F. Conti, MD
Fabiana Q. Silva, MD
Rishi P. Singh, MD

Postoperative pseudophakic macular edema (PME) is the accumulation of extracellular fluid with anatomical alteration of the macula after cataract surgery. The pathogenesis of PME is multifactorial; however, the major etiology seems to be inflammatory mediators released in the aqueous and vitreous humors after surgical manipulation. Inflammation breaks down the blood-aqueous and blood-retinal barriers, leading to increased retinal vascular permeability. Postoperative PME is the most frequent complication following cataract extraction and usually presents 4 to 6 weeks after surgery, with a reported range of 3 weeks to 6 months. It can be found in up to 81% of patients on postoperative optical coherence tomography (OCT). Nevertheless, clinical PME following phacoemulsification is much less common (0.1% to 2.35%). Surgical risk factors are intra- and extracapsular cataract extractions, posterior capsule rupture, zonular dialysis, retained lens fragments, and vitreous loss. Preexisting risk factors are the presence of epiretinal membrane, diabetic retinopathy, history of uveitis, previous retinal venous occlusion, and retinal detachment repair.[1]

With regard to prevention of macular edema in the postoperative period, many surgeons use postoperative topical non-steroidal anti-inflammatory drugs (NSAIDs) and steroids prophylactically, especially in high-risk patients. The first evidence that this was a valid treatment approach came from a recent multicenter, randomized, double-masked study of 263 adult diabetic patients with nonproliferative diabetic retinopathy requiring cataract surgery.[2] This study demonstrated that a significantly lower percentage of patients that used nepafenac before surgery developed macular edema when compared to patients in the placebo group (3.2% vs 16.7%; $P < 0.001$).[2]

The diagnosis of postoperative PME is confirmed by fluorescein angiography (FA) (Figure 30-1) and OCT (Figure 30-2). Postoperative PME can also be called *Irvine-Gass syndrome* when

Fekrat S, ed. *Curbside Consultation in Retina: 49 Clinical Questions, Second Edition.* (pp 153-155).
© 2019 SLACK Incorporated

Figure 30-1. FA showing hyperfluorescence of the disc and petaloid leakage in the macula consistent with PME.

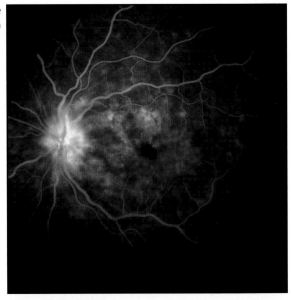

Figure 30-2. OCT image showing postoperative cystoid macular edema.

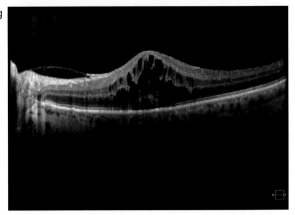

macular edema is accompanied by optic nerve head hyperfluorescence and leakage on FA. OCT is useful in identifying macular thickening, cystic spaces, and occasionally subfoveal fluid. OCT is also valuable in recognizing subclinical vitreomacular traction and epiretinal membranes, which may complicate the diagnosis of postoperative PME.[3]

Once the diagnosis is confirmed, initial treatment includes topical NSAIDs and topical corticosteroids. A double-masked, prospective trial of 28 patients that evaluated clinical cystoid macular edema after cataract extraction demonstrated that patients treated with combination therapy of ketorolac and prednisolone were more likely to experience recovery of 2 lines or more of visual acuity than patients treated with monotherapy with either agent alone (prednisolone 50%, ketorolac 67%, combination 89%; $P < 0.001$).[4] The use of peri- and intraocular steroids injections for postoperative PME is supported by several case series. Triesence (triamcinolone acetate) was the first preservative-free steroid approved for intraocular use and has subsequently been used for the management of macular edema. Kenalog (triamcinolone) administered into the sub-Tenon space can also be used to treat PME. Proper placement in the sub-Tenon space nearest to the macula is essential in order to achieve the maximum response to the drug; however, there are potential complications, including elevated intraocular pressure (IOP) and risk of infections. Other valuable options to consider are long-acting steroid delivery systems, such as the Ozurdex implant (dexamethasone). It can be inserted into the vitreous cavity, producing a long-lasting anti-inflammatory effect (4 to 6 months) and a more tolerable IOP variation.[5] Corticosteroid use has to be balanced against the high rate of side effects, the most common being the increase in IOP. Typically, there is good treatment effect with edema reduction on OCT and leakage improvement on FA.

Anti-vascular endothelial growth factor (anti-VEGF) antibodies, including bevacizumab, ranibizumab, and aflibercept, may also be a valuable option for the treatment of postoperative PME. While not commonly used to treat postoperative PME, several case series demonstrated its utility in improving visual acuity and OCT findings. It is important to note, however, that intra- and periocular steroid injections as well as intravitreal anti-VEGF agents are not approved by the Food and Drug Administration for PME treatment. In patients unresponsive to medical treatment, Pendergast et al[6,7] presented a retrospective analysis of 23 patients with chronic PME who underwent pars plana vitrectomy, resulting in macular edema resolution with improved visual acuity in approximately 70% of cases.

In our experience, treatment starts with a topical NSAID, either prior to surgery or when operative risk factors are identified, to minimize or even attempt to prevent postoperative PME development. If postoperative PME is diagnosed, we start a topical NSAID (ie, kerotolac, diclofencac, nepafenac, bromfenac) in combination with a topical steroid (ie, prednisolone) unless contraindicated. It can typically take 6 to 12 weeks to achieve improvement in visual acuity, contrast sensitivity, and leakage on FA. Even cases of long-term PME (> 6 months) can respond to topical therapy alone. Generally, we defer intravitreal steroids injections in favor of topical therapy for at least 6 weeks. Follow-up OCTs are needed to document change. If no improvement is achieved with topical treatment, then intravitreal steroids, instead of periocular, are considered. The macular edema resolution can last for up to 3 months, and the procedure may be repeated if needed. Intravitreal anti-VEGF agents are only used in patients with glaucoma or with a previous history of steroid-induced ocular hypertension. In the minority of cases when postoperative PME does not resolve spontaneously after topical or intravitreal treatment, we have performed pars plana vitrectomy with elevation of the posterior hyaloid as a last resort.

References

1. Chu CJ, Johnston RL, Buscombe C, et al; United Kingdom Pseudophakic Macular Edema Study Group. Risk factors and incidence of macular edema after cataract surgery: a database study of 81984 eyes. *Ophthalmology.* 2016;123(2):316-323.
2. Singh R, Alpern L, Jaffe GJ, et al. Evaluation of nepafenac in prevention of macular edema following cataract surgery in patients with diabetic retinopathy. *Clin Ophthalmol.* 2012;6:1259-1269.
3. Guo S, Patel S, Baumrind B, et al. Management of pseudophakic cystoid macular edema. *Surv Ophthalmol.* 2015;60(2):123-137.
4. Heier JS, Topping TM, Baumann W, Dirks MS, Chern S. Ketorolac versus prednisolone versus combination therapy in the treatment of acute pseudophakic cystoid macular edema. *Ophthalmology.* 2000;107(11):2034-2038.
5. Mayer WJ, Kurz S, Wolf A, et al. Dexamethasone implant as an effective treatment option for macular edema due to Irvine-Gass syndrome. *J Cataract Refract Surg.* 2015;41(9):1954-1961.
6. Pendergast SD, Hassan TS, Williams GA, et al. Vitrectomy for diffuse diabetic macular edema associated with a taut premacular posterior hyaloid. *Am J Ophthalmol.* 2000:130(2):178-186.
7. Pendergast SD, Margherio RR, Williams GA, Cox MS. Vitrectomy for chronic pseudophakic cystoid macular edema. *Am J Ophthalmol.* 1999;128(3):317-323.

WHAT IS DYELESS ANGIOGRAPHY (OPTICAL COHERENCE TOMOGRAPHY ANGIOGRAPHY) AND WHAT DO I NEED I KNOW ABOUT IT? WILL IT REPLACE FLUORESCEIN ANGIOGRAPHY?

Thomas Hwang, MD
Yali Jia, PhD

Optical coherence tomography (OCT) has revolutionized the management of retinal diseases by providing high-resolution, 3-dimensional (3D) structural images of the retina rapidly and noninvasively. OCT angiography (OCT-A) visualizes blood flow by obtaining OCT images at the exact same place sequentially and analyzing the difference between the images caused by the moving blood cells. This difference is called *decorrelation* or *variance* in the amplitude or phase of the OCT wave signal. Dense, contiguous images are then stitched together to create a volume that contains structural and flow information in 3D. These volumes are then segmented according to laminar structures and displayed in *en face* orientation to display angiograms, creating images that are analogous to fluorescein angiography (FA). These segmented volumes are called *slabs*. OCT angiograms can be presented in cross-sectional orientation, same as OCT B-scans, with colors to show where the flow is to demonstrate its relationship to the anatomical structures.

Currently available commercial systems include AngioVue (Optovue) and AngioPlex (Zeiss), which are high-speed spectral domain OCT systems (~70,000 axials scans/second). Commercial swept source OCT systems with 100,000 axial scans or faster are planned. Without need for a dye injection, angiographic images can be produced in a few seconds. The available field of view include 3x3 mm, 4.5x4.5 mm, 6x6 mm, and 8x8 mm. Capillary details are best seen on 3x3 mm angiograms. The standard output presents 4 slabs: superficial and deep retinal plexuses; the outer retina, which is normally avascular but where choroidal neovascularization (CNV) would be found; and the choriocapillaris (Figure 31-1).

The retinal vasculature is known to have up to 4 distinct layers. Around the optic disc, the radial peripapillary capillaries are found in the nerve fiber layer. In the macula, 3 distinct vascular

Fekrat S, ed. *Curbside Consultation in Retina: 49 Clinical Questions, Second Edition.* (pp 157-160).
© 2019 SLACK Incorporated

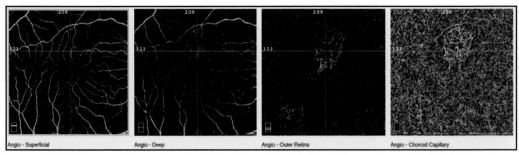

Figure 31-1. Commercial output of OCT-A of a patient with CNV associated with punctate inner choroidopathy. The superficial slab shows normal retinal vasculature. The deep slab shows significant projection artifacts from the superficial slab. The outer retina shows the CNV, which casts a projection artifact onto the choroid capillary slab.

Figure 31-2. OCT-A shows an area of CNV in yellow (C), seen as occult CNV on FA (B). A cross sectional angiogram (D) shows that CNV is under the retinal pigment epithelium. (Reprinted with permission from Jia Y, Bailey ST, Hwang TS, et al. Quantitative OCT-A of vascular abnormalities in the living human eye. *Proc Natl Acad Sci USA.* 2015;112(18):E2395-E2402. doi:10.1073/pnas.1500185112.)

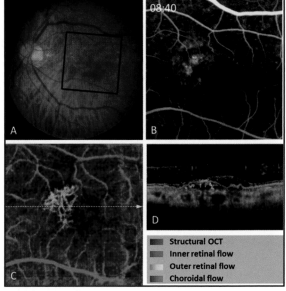

plexuses are seen. The superficial vascular complex resides mainly in the ganglion cell layer and consists of the branching vessels that we are familiar with from FA. Two deeper capillary networks that flank the inner nuclear layer are called intermediate and deep capillary plexuses. These are networks of anastomosing capillaries of uniform density and caliber. They merge into a single layer in the midperiphery. At the foveal avascular zone edge, the capillaries from all 3 retinal vascular plexuses merge into a single layer. A distinct vascular network called the *radial peripapillary capillary plexus* can be found in the nerve fiber layer of the region near the optic disc. The current commercial output treats the intermediate and deep capillary plexus as a single plexuses and refers to it as *deep plexus*. Generally, FA only visualizes the superficial vascular complex. OCT-A can visualize all layers of the retinal vasculature.[1]

In addition to visualizing vasculature not visible with FA, OCT-A can present vascular information in the context of the structural information in 3D. Vessels above the internal limiting membrane can be unambiguously identified as retinal neovascularization. CNV can be diagnosed by their location between the outer plexiform layer and Bruch membrane (Figure 31-2). This is especially valuable in conditions where dye leakage is present without neovascularization, such as central serous chorioretinopathy or Type II macular telangiectasia, where FA interpretation can be ambiguous. OCT-A can also demonstrate capillary nonperfusion, microaneurysms, arteriolar narrowing, and dilation of vessels.[2] Vascular nonperfusion, dilation, and vessel density can be automatically quantified as potentially useful biomarkers because OCT-A has higher contrast than FA and is never affected by leakage. However, OCT-A does not reveal dynamic information, such as transit time and vascular permeability.[3]

Understanding artifacts specific to OCT-A is critical in the proper interpretation of the images. First is motion artifact, because detecting motion with high sensitivity is how OCT-A works, motion from anything besides blood flow (eg, microsaccades and blinks) can disrupt and degrade image quality. Motion artifacts look like bright lines, vertical or horizontal, and can interfere with interpretation of the images. While approaches such as eye tracking and orthogonal registration and merging of images have been successful in reducing these artifacts, residual motion artifacts are common and excellent patient cooperation is critical in obtaining high quality images.

Second is projection artifacts. The moving blood cells in the superficial vasculature cast a moving shadow in the deeper tissues, resulting in a decorrelation signal in the deeper tissue. This results in a cast of the superficial vasculature in the deeper slab angiogram, interfering with its interpretation. Because this artifact has a tail shape axially, the layers of the vasculature blur into the deeper layer making segmentation difficult. This is one reason that commercial systems present the retinal vasculature as 2 layers, although the histologic studies have shown that there are 3 distinct layers.

Several approaches have been tried to reduce these artifacts. One is slab subtraction, where the cast of superficial vascular pattern is used to erase the projected pattern in the deep plexus angiograms. While it eliminates the positive artifacts, it also disrupts the real vessels and makes the interpretation of the deep plexus angiogram difficult. Another is to find a thin slab in the deeper plexus that has less projection artifact. This approach is a manual process and employed in some published studies, but may be impractical in day-to-day clinical use. Another is to move the boundary of segmentation to be more posterior to avoid the most intense projection artifact and present a more distinctly different vascular pattern.[4] Finally, Zhang and colleagues[5] have described an algorithm that resolves the ambiguity between true flow and projection-induced decorrelation. This approach has allowed segmentation of the macular retinal plexus into 3 distinct layers according to known anatomic boundaries and produces clean angiograms of the deeper plexuses.

Summary

OCT-A is an exciting new technology that shows capillary level details of the retinal vasculature without the need for dye injection. Its 3D capabilities and high contrast allow for quantification and automatic detection of pathology, which may prove to be an important tool in the management of retinal vascular diseases. Although OCT-A has clear advantages over FA, it is important to remember that FA was foundational to many landmark clinical trials and the findings on OCT-A and FA may not be equivalent. Also, the current field of view on OCT-A is significantly less than those of FA. Understanding the differences between the technologies as well as the artifacts and limitations that are specific to OCT-A will allow us to adopt this new technology without losing wisdom from the old.

References

1. Campbell JP, Zhang M, Hwang TS, et al. Detailed vascular anatomy of the human retina by projection- resolved optical coherence tomography angiography. *Nature*. 2017;7:1-11. doi: 10.1038/srep42201
2. Hwang TS, Zhang M, Bhavsar K, et al. Visualization of 3 distinct retinal plexuses by projection-resolved optical coherence tomography angiography in diabetic retinopathy. *JAMA Ophthalmol*. 2016;134(12):1411-1419. doi: 10.1001/jamaophthalmol.2016.4272
3. Jia Y, Bailey ST, Hwang TS, et al. Quantitative optical coherence tomography angiography of vascular abnormalities in the living human eye. *Proc Natl Acad Sci USA*. 2015;112(18):E2395-E2402. doi: 10.1073/pnas.1500185112
4. Spaide RF, Fujimoto JG, Waheed NK. Image artifacts in optical coherence tomography angiography. *Retina*. 2015;35(11):2163-2180. doi: 10.1097/IAE.0000000000000765
5. Zhang M, Hwang TS, Campbell JP, et al. Projection-resolved optical coherence tomographic angiography. *Biomed Opt Express*. 2016;7(3):816–13. doi: 10.1364/BOE.7.000816

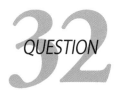

QUESTION

CENTRAL SEROUS? WHAT NOW? MANAGEMENT OPTIONS FOR CENTRAL SEROUS RETINOPATHY

Lisa C. Olmos de Koo, MD, MBA

First, take a deep breath and try to stay calm (this goes for both the treating physician and the patient). Second, carefully revisit your diagnosis by reviewing the clinical history and imaging studies. Central serous retinopathy (CSR), also known as *central serous chorioretinopathy*, is a chorioretinal disease that can have a chronic and relapsing course, characterized by the accumulation of subretinal fluid (SRF) in the posterior pole as well as pigment epithelial detachments (PEDs). The exact pathophysiology of this unique condition remains obscure, although retinal pigment epithelial (RPE) dysfunction and hyperpermeability of choroidal vessels are thought to contribute. Hypercortisolic states (eg, external stressors, exogenous steroid administration) may also play a role in triggering episodes in predisposed individuals.

The demographic group most commonly affected by CSR is healthy males in young to middle adulthood. However, CSR has been reported in adults of all age groups and does not appear to have a strong racial or ethnic predisposition. In the past, the frequency of this condition may have been underestimated prior to the era of widespread use of optical coherence tomography (OCT). The classic exam features of CSR include well-circumscribed serous retinal detachments as well as serous PEDs, which are evident on spectral domain OCT (Figure 32-1). Patches of RPE disruption and PEDs, representing resolved acute episodes, are often detected upon careful examination of the fellow eye, as the condition is commonly bilateral. Fundus autofluorescence can be useful in these cases, sometimes demonstrating dependent atrophic RPE tracks. Increased subfoveal choroidal thickness (pachychoroid) in both eyes is another feature that can be seen on enhanced depth imaging OCT.[1] Fluorescein angiography (FA) is not required to establish the diagnosis, but it can be helpful in atypical cases and is required for planning photodynamic therapy (PDT), as discussed later. Classic FA patterns include the expansile dot, smokestack, and diffuse patterns

Fekrat S, ed. *Curbside Consultation in Retina: 49 Clinical Questions, Second Edition.* (pp 161-166).
© 2019 SLACK Incorporated

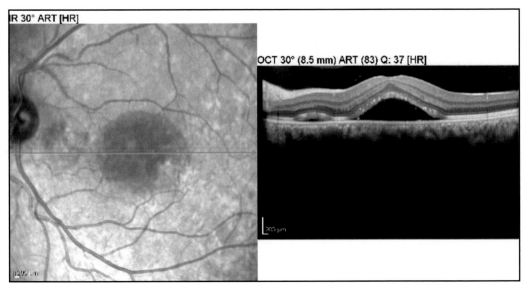

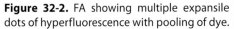

Figure 32-1. Spectral domain OCT showing the classic features of CSR with a well-circumscribed pocket of subfoveal fluid.

Figure 32-2. FA showing multiple expansile dots of hyperfluorescence with pooling of dye.

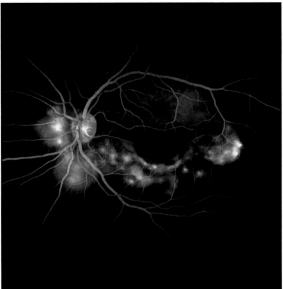

of hyperfluorescence (Figure 32-2). Indocyanine green angiography demonstrates choroidal hyperpermeability. More recently characterized OCT angiographic findings include increased choroidal vascular flow.[2]

It is important to distinguish the findings of acute CSR from choroidal neovascularization (CNV) because the optimal treatment for these conditions is distinct. Intraretinal fluid or sub-retinal tissue on OCT and/or hemorrhage noted on fundus exam should prompt consideration of CNV, which may even be secondary to chronic CSR (Figure 32-3). Patients with CNV should be treated promptly with intravitreal anti-vascular endothelial growth factor (anti-VEGF) therapy. Along the same lines, the onset of newly diagnosed CSR over the age of 60 should raise a red flag for CNV and both eyes should be closely evaluated for subtle findings of age-related macular

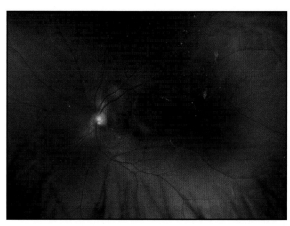

Figure 32-3. Color fundus photo of the left eye of a patient with known chronic CSR. New subretinal hemorrhage is a clue that this patient has developed secondary CNV.

degeneration (AMD). Coexistence of CSR and CNV is possible, especially in cases of chronic, untreated CSR or in older patients. Interestingly, chronic CSR has been associated with the same genetic variants implicated in AMD, but the alleles that confer risk for one condition may be protective for the other, and vice versa.[3] There is clearly still much to be learned about the overlap between these 2 conditions.

Once the diagnosis of CSR is established, your first role as the treating physician is to counsel and reassure the patient as well as to establish a schedule of regular monitoring exams. CSR patients appreciate thoughtful counseling about the diagnosis and prognosis. It is helpful to let them know that most patients (90%) recover 20/30 or better visual acuity; however, recurrences occur in 30% to 50%. This potential for recurrence and the bilateral nature of the condition should be discussed, as well as the need to present to the clinic for evaluation and imaging whenever new symptoms are noticed. I usually ask my chronic CSR patients to try to present for evaluation within 2 weeks of the onset of a new symptomatic episode. This becomes especially important over the age of 55, as secondary CNV is more common in this age group.

Avoidance of exogenous steroids is important for CSR patients, as steroids can trigger acute episodes. Steroids may sensitize the eye to adrenergic hormones that in turn may cause choriocapillaris hyperpermeability and RPE cellular degeneration.[4] In addition to oral steroids, other often-overlooked steroid sources include inhalers or nasal sprays (eg, those prescribed for asthma or allergies), intra-articular injections (often administered by our orthopedic colleagues), or even topical preparations used for various dermatologic conditions. I like to ask my patients specifically about exposure to any of these steroid preparations, and I review their medication list in detail, including over-the-counter supplements and herbal preparations. When in doubt, ask patients to discontinue supplements whose contents cannot be identified. When I establish a new CSR diagnosis, I usually prepare a letter for the patient's primary care physician (PCP) requesting avoidance of exogenous steroid whenever possible. In certain medical conditions (eg, asthma, organ transplants, autoimmune or connective tissue disorders), steroids are a mainstay of therapy. In these cases, I communicate with the PCP to ensure that any option for steroid-sparing agents has been considered. If steroid avoidance is not possible, earlier therapy for subfoveal fluid may be indicated. Other medications, such as exogenous testosterone, can also be potential triggers. The complexities of the endocrine interplay in this condition are, as yet, incompletely understood.

Acute CSR has also been associated with increased endogenous cortisol. Ask your CSR patients about their life stressors and take the time listen for a few minutes; you may be surprised by what you hear. Then, ask what kind of things they do to manage their stress level. I encourage my CSR patients to engage in at least 20 minutes a day of a healthy activity of their choosing to distract them from life's responsibilities and stresses. For many, exercise is extremely effective, whether it be a walk outside after dinner or a brisk run in the morning before work. For some, dedicated time to rest and relax is more effective.

After the initial diagnosis of an acute episode of CSR-related SRF, I usually give a follow-up appointment in approximately 1 month. I generally follow these patients monthly with serial OCTs until I observe complete resolution of macular SRF. Associated PEDs will often, but not always, persist. Of note, these patients can also have extramacular pockets of SRF. I do not follow these closely, because their persistence or resolution will not impact central vision to a measurable degree. At the 2-month mark after initial diagnosis, if I see no decrease in the height of subfoveal fluid or other sign of resolution, I usually begin discussing therapeutic options with the patient. This is a good time to reinitiate contact with the PCP and request that a basic chemistry panel and liver function tests be drawn in preparation for possible medical therapy. If there is no PCP, I do request that they establish care with one at this point. If SRF persists and has not decreased at the 3-month mark from initial presentation or symptom onset, I will generally offer therapy. Therapeutic options for CSR today can be divided into local and systemic.

Laser for chronic CSR is an effective local treatment option. Today, thermal laser is less frequently used than in the past due to the availability of other treatment options as well as the potential for scarring that can result in paracentral scotoma or secondary CNV. However, it can still play a useful role when leakage sites are far from the foveal center and a more permanent solution is desired. These patients can develop new areas of leak after thermal laser, but the site that was treated typically does not leak again. PDT or *cold laser* is currently preferred over thermal laser and has been proven safe and effective for chronic CSR as well as for acute CSR when more rapid visual rehabilitation is desired.[5-7] It has also proven effective for steroid-associated CSR.[8] PDT using verteporfin addresses choroidal hyperpermeability by focally reinforcing the RPE's blood-retinal barrier and has been shown to resolve SRF in over 80% of patients. Verteporfin has a high affinity for abnormal blood vessels and when stimulated by a 689 nm nonthermal light, it produces highly reactive short-lived oxygen radicals, resulting in the selective damage of the dysfunctional blood vessels. This treatment requires intravenous access for both the treatment planning FA and the verteporfin infusion, as well as protection from UV light for 48 to 72 hours post-therapy. The laser spot size should be set to about 1000 μm greater than the area of maximal leakage at 5 minutes on the FA. If there are multiple spots of leakage, one may try to encompass these areas in a single larger spot, or repeat the therapy in a different spot after the first delivery, with first priority to the spot that is closest to the fovea. Reduced fluence settings (300 mW/cm², 25 J/cm², 83 seconds) may be used with success. After treatment, monitor for SRF resolution at around 4 to 6 weeks post-therapy. Late recurrences at the treated leaking point(s) are common and can be safely retreated as early as 3 months after the initial treatment. Complications of PDT for CSR are rare but include acute severe vision decrease in 1.5%. Finally, subthreshold micropulse laser has also been utilized with reported success in the literature, but at present its use is not uniformly widespread in the United States.[9]

Another local therapy for CSR, intravitreal anti-VEGF therapy, is more controversial. There is a mechanistic rationale for the use of this therapy given that these agents decrease vascular permeability, including that of the choriocapillaris. Clinical efficacy has also been demonstrated via several studies and reports in the literature.[10] However, clinically the robustness of the therapeutic response to anti-VEGF agents in CSR is less than in CNV or macular edema due to retinal venous occlusion or diabetic retinopathy. Personally, I do not employ anti-VEGF as a first-line therapy for CSR. One important exception is those patients in whom I see evidence of secondary CNV formation, namely intraretinal fluid, subretinal tissue, or frank hemorrhage (see Figure 32-2). In these cases, I advocate treatment of the CNV with careful attention to CSR if it is also present in the fellow eye.

Oral systemic medical therapy for CSR has garnered much attention in the literature in recent years, and it may be favored over local therapy for a variety of patient-specific reasons.[11] Personally, I find that medical therapy can be a useful option, especially for patients who have multiple leaking spots in whom laser delivery is more complex. I have also found that systemic agents can be very helpful in the bullous variant of CSR. There are 2 main classes of medications that can be used effectively to treat CSR: metabolism inducers (eg, rifampin) and endogenous mineralocorticoid receptor antagonists (eg, eplerenone, spironolactone). The choice between systemic agents may be informed by their different side effect profiles, as discussed later. Given their mechanisms of action, however, systemic medications are not the optimal choice for CSR patients who depend upon steroid treatments to prevent transplant rejection or to maintain quiescence in chronic inflammatory conditions. Rather, these patients are generally best served by local therapy, such as PDT.[8] It is important to inform patients that the use of any oral medication for CSR is off-label, and that there is no US Food and Drug Administration–approved treatment for the condition at the present time. As always, consultation and partnership with the patient's PCP is recommended.

Eplerenone (Inspra) appears to work via the antagonism of specific mineralocorticoid receptors that would normally allow corticosteroid binding to trigger choroidal vasodilation and contribute to hyperpermeability.[12] Eplerenone's most common side effect is hyperkalemia, necessitating caution in patients with diabetes or renal failure. I usually check a chemistry panel prior to initiation, at 1 month postinitiation, and every 6 months thereafter while on therapy. 50 mg orally daily is the standard dose. Some patients may wish to start at 25 mg daily and ramp up to the full dose after several weeks on therapy. I monitor monthly for resolution and will consider discontinuation after full resolution for 1 month. In cases of relapse, I may consider maintenance dosing of 25 mg daily, which is generally well-tolerated. Spironolactone acts via a similar mechanism of mineralocorticoid receceptor antagnoism; however, it is generally less well tolerated than eplerenone due to the potential for gynecomastia. It is also significantly less expensive, making it more accessible.

Rifampin (Rifadin) is an antibiotic whose mechanism of action in the setting of CSR is induction of the cytochrome P450 pathway to metabolize endogenous or exogenous corticosteroids. It is thus necessary to check liver function tests before initiating treatment. It is also prudent to monitor the liver function tests 1 month after initiating therapy and successively every 3 months if chronic therapy is needed. I also ask patients to abstain from any alcohol intake while on this medication. Rifampin's effectiveness at treating CSR was first discovered in a patient being concurrently treated for *Mycobacterium avium intracellulare*. One recent study showed complete response in nearly half of eyes treated with rifampin, including those who had failed other forms of therapy.[13] Personally, I prescribe a dose of 300 mg orally daily, and I recommend follow-up monthly with serial OCTs until the fluid has resolved. If fluid does resolve, I discontinue therapy. I do not recommend maintenance therapy with this particular medication due to the rare potential for severe side effects. If there is no reduction in fluid after the first month of therapy, I may consider increasing the dose. If no effect is seen 1 month after 600 mg daily, I generally discontinue the therapy. Side effects of rifampin range from rashes, gastrointestinal upset, and flu-like symptoms to serious and rare complications such as hepatitis and Stevens-Johnson syndrome.

Rarely, some patients with the bullous variant of CSR who develop extensive serous retinal detachments ultimately require repair using vitreoretinal surgical techniques including scleral buckle and vitrectomy with intraocular tamponade. In these cases, care should be taken to exclude treatable diagnoses such as infection or occult neoplasm, and biopsy with analysis of intraocular fluid is warranted at the time of surgery.

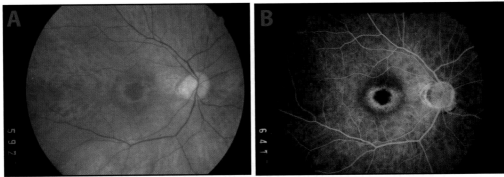

Figure 33-1. (A, B) Hydroxychloroquine maculopathy in a typical bull's eye pattern in a patient being treated for rheumatoid arthritis. The fluorescein angiogram (FA) documents a transmission defect corresponding to the area of pigment alteration. The visual acuity was 20/60.

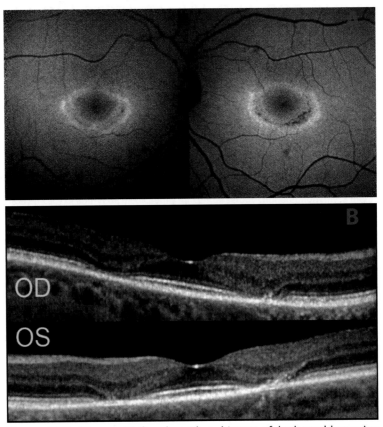

Figure 33-2. 53-year-old female with a history of hydroxychloroquine therapy for 17 years for Sjogren syndrome, with an approximate cumulative dose of 1.6 kg. (A) Fundus autofluorescence of the right and left eyes demonstrating a typical band of perifoveal hyperautofluorescence in both eyes. (B) OCT of the right and left eyes demonstrating significant perifoveal outer retinal and ellipsoid segment attenuation in both eyes.

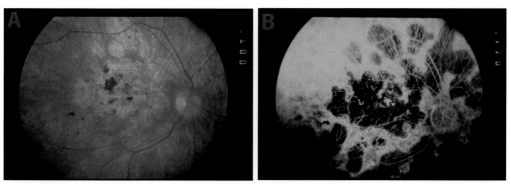

Figure 33-3. (A, B) Thioridazine toxicity in a geographic nummular pattern. The FA documents geographic loss of RPE and choriocapillaris. The visual acuity was 20/200.

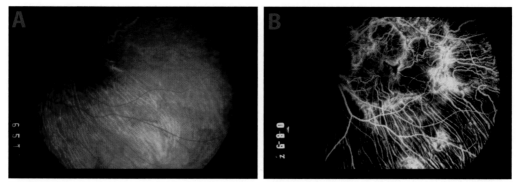

Figure 33-4. (A, B) Advanced thioridazine toxicity resembling retinitis pigmentosa. The FA reveals virtually complete loss of RPE, allowing for visualization of the larger choroidal vessels. The visual acuity was hand motion.

taken seriously. Multifocal electroretinography can be particularly helpful for confirming early toxicity and monitoring recovery, commonly exhibiting diminished wave amplitudes in the parafoveal region when toxicity is present. Retinal toxicity may occur in a more perifoveal than parafoveal distribution in Asian patients. If hydroxychloroquine toxicity is suspected, typically medication discontinuation is recommended; however, retinal changes may persist or even worsen after cessation of drug therapy.

Mellaril (thioridazine) is an antipsychotic drug that was once widely utilized; however, because of concern of significant retinal toxicity, it currently is less frequently prescribed. From the retinal standpoint, it is one of the most toxic medications. A daily dosage greater than 800 mg/day can cause considerable retinal damage, though when utilized at a lower dosage there is less concern. Acute toxicity may present with a variable degree of central visual impairment, dyschromatopsia, and nyctalopia. Early fundus abnormalities include granular pigment stippling, which can readily progress to circumscribed areas of RPE and choriocapillaris loss, often in a nummular pattern (Figure 33-3).[3] Photography and FA are useful ancillary tests. FA highlights the initial irregularity of the RPE followed by severe atrophy of the choriocapillaris in the late stages of disease (Figure 33-4). Visual fields, electroretinography, and electrooculography may be variably effective but are not good screening tools. If evidence of toxicity is discovered, the medication should be promptly discontinued. Progressive retinal changes may occur for years because the medication is indefinitely stored in the eye.

Nolvadex (tamoxifen), an estrogen antagonist, is used in the treatment of breast adenocarcinoma and advanced glioblastoma multiforme. Despite early descriptions of crystalline retinopathy

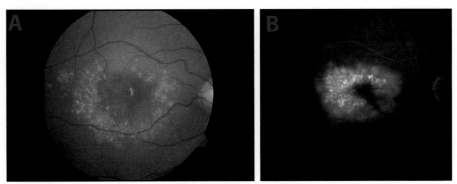

Figure 33-5. (A, B) Tamoxifen crystalline retinopathy. Yellowish-white intraretinal crystalline deposits are seen in a perifoveal distribution. There is prominent underlying cystoid macular edema (CME). (Reprinted with permission from David Sarraf.)

at high doses (60 to 100 mg/day), toxicity is unusual at doses of 20 mg/day or less, although crystals may still be seen in 3% to 4% with chronic administration. Early symptoms include mild decreased vision and dyschromatopsia. Clinically, yellowish-white intraretinal crystalline deposits are noted, usually in a parafoveal distribution (Figure 33-5).[4] Other associated features include corneal verticillata, retinal pigmentary changes, and CME. OCT may reveal hyperreflective inner plexiform deposits, photoreceptor disruption, and CME. Despite crystalline deposition, there is typically little change in retinal function, and asymptomatic patients are generally monitored, as the medication is needed for treatment of the underlying malignancy. However, if there is confirmed evidence of retinal dysfunction, then consideration should be given to discontinue the medication and replacement with other estrogen antagonists.

Viagra (sildenafil), as well as other selective phosphodiesterase-5 inhibitors, are commonly prescribed for male erectile dysfunction. Although selective for the penile corpora cavernosa, cross-reactivity with phosphodiesterase-6 in photoreceptors occurs and may be responsible for ocular changes. Bluish dyschromatopsia, halos, and increased light sensitivity lasting minutes to hours may occur after ingesting the lowest therapeutic dose (25 mg/day). These symptoms occur more frequently at higher doses (100 mg/day). Reports describing objective findings are uncommon but include retinal hemorrhages, retinal vascular occlusion, acceleration of proliferative diabetic retinopathy, oculomotor nerve palsy, central serous chorioretinopathy, and nonarteritic anterior ischemic optic neuropathy (NAION).[5] There are no recognized long-term toxic effects following chronic administration of the medication, although patients who have experienced NAION in one eye should be discouraged from using sildenafil, as it may potentiate the risk of developing NAION in the fellow eye. There is no indication for routine screening at this time, but counseling patients with preexisting retinal disease is prudent, and symptomatic patients should be evaluated for retinal pathology.

Summary

Although there are thousands of systemic medications, only a small number of these agents produce retinal changes. Retinal toxicity can occur when agents are used at standard therapeutic dosages or when utilized for non-approved indications. With multiple new drugs reaching the market annually, ophthalmologists need to maintain a high index of suspicion that patients' clinical findings and visual symptoms may be related to one or more of their systemic medications.

References

1. Marmor MF, Kellner U, Lai TY, Melles RB, Mieler WF; American Academy of Ophthalmology. Recommendations on screening for chloroquine and hydroxychloroquine retinopathy (2016 revision). *Ophthalmology.* 2016;123(6):1386-1394.
2. Rodriguez-Padilla JA, Hedges TR III, Monson B, et al. High-speed ultra-high-resolution optical coherence tomography findings in hydroxychloroquine retinopathy. *Arch Ophthalmol.* 2007;125(6):775-780.
3. Meredith TA, Aaberg TM, Willerson WD. Progressive chorioretinopathy after receiving thioridazine. *Arch Ophthalmol.* 1978;96(7):1172-1176.
4. Kaiser-Kupfer MI, Kupfer C, Rodrigues MM. Tamoxifen retinopathy. A clinicopathologic report. *Ophthalmology.* 1981;88(1):89-93.
5. Vobig MA. Retinal side-effects of sildenafil. *Lancet.* 1999;353(9162):1442.

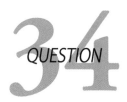

SHOULD I SEND A PATIENT WITH A LARGE CHRONIC MACULAR HOLE TO A RETINA DOCTOR? DO THEY EVEN OPERATE ON THOSE?

Avni P. Finn, MD, MBA

Tamer H. Mahmoud, MD, PhD

Yes, we do! Macular hole repair is a very successful surgery and most full-thickness macular holes close with conventional surgery involving vitrectomy, internal limiting membrane (ILM) peeling, and the use of gas tamponade. Nevertheless, about 10% of macular holes fail to close with this technique.[1]

Large macular holes are defined by the International Vitreomacular Traction Study group as those that are more than 400 μm in diameter. Chronic holes are those present for longer than 6 months based on history. Large chronic macular holes present a surgical challenge for the vitreoretinal surgeon, but one that may be tackled with various newer surgical techniques. While some of these will close with the conventional technique, others do not and may have higher rates of recurrence, such as those macular holes associated with high myopia, retinal detachment, trauma, and juxtafoveal telangiectasia. A combination of different techniques have been employed to improve closure rates in these difficult macular holes, including scleral shortening techniques, macular buckles, inverted or free ILM flaps, autologous lens capsular flaps, autologous retinal transplant, and the use of adjuvant blood components.

Scleral Shortening Techniques

Highly myopic patients with full-thickness macular holes present a unique challenge. They often have thin, brittle ILM that is difficult to peel. The retina in these patients is stretched thin, with schisis or foveal detachment accompanying the hole. In highly myopic eyes, scleral

Fekrat S. *Curbside Consultation in Retina: 49 Clinical
Questions, Second Edition.* (pp 173-176).
© 2019 SLACK Incorporated

shortening techniques have been used to decrease the degree of curvature of the eye and reduce the posterior staphyloma, thereby decreasing tractional forces on the retina and providing less surface area for the retina to cover along the posterior pole to allow holes to close. This technique was initially described using scleral resection but has since evolved to scleral imbrication whereby mattress sutures are placed in the temporal equatorial sclera, which imbricate the temporal sclera as they are tightened.[2] While this process shortens the axial length and decreases the staphyloma, it is likely that vitrectomy and ILM peeling are the more crucial steps in closing the macular hole.

Scleral buckling for myopic macular holes is an old technique that has gained some renewed interest with newer buckling devices that may be safer and easier to use in pathologic myopes with macular hole, posterior staphyloma, and retinal detachment. In this technique, a specialized rubber radial element with a terminal plate designed to infold the macula is placed to decrease the stretching effect of the posterior staphyloma.[3] Vitrectomy and ILM peeling are usually performed concurrently with the macular buckle. Effective and safe placement of the macular buckle remains a concern with this technique. Additionally, given postoperative complications, including subretinal and choroidal hemorrhage, erosion, diplopia, and focal retinal pigment epithelium atrophy, we favor the use of other techniques described.

Autologous Internal Limiting Membrane Flap

The initial report of the inverted ILM flap technique for a large macular hole was performed by peeling the ILM around the macular hole and leaving the central part of the ILM in place and inverting this to cover the macular hole.[4] Various modifications have since been made to this technique, including peeling the ILM on only the temporal side of the fovea and covering the macular hole with a temporal ILM flap. Other groups have described peeling a free flap the same size as the macular hole and placing this inside the macular hole. As the ILM flap can be very flimsy and difficult to maneuver, injecting viscoelastic over the flap to secure it in place or adjusting the flap under perfluorocarbon may be useful adjuncts to this technique. In our experience, ILM flaps are most successfully used in patients with myopic macular holes.

The ILM flap acts as a scaffold for Müller cell and tissue proliferation. An inverted ILM flap is thought to induce glial cell proliferation. These proliferating glial cells then provide an environment suitable for photoreceptors to migrate to the fovea, explaining the improvement in vision. On optical coherence tomography, anatomic improvements are seen in the foveal contour, and there is some restoration of the ellipsoid zone and external limiting membrane.

Lens Capsule Flap

The lens capsule has recently been described as an alternative tissue scaffold. An anterior capsular flap can be harvested after the anterior capsulotomy in phakic patients or a posterior capsular flap can be harvested in a pseudophakic patient. The anterior capsule is thicker and more rigid than the flimsy posterior capsule, making it easier to maneuver into the macular hole and less likely to scroll in the hole. These flaps cannot be used when there is limited capsular material to harvest, such as in pseudophakic eyes with a prior posterior capsulotomy.[5] The transparency of the tissue makes it difficult to see and manipulate during this procedure unless it is stained with a vital dye. Additionally, there is an increased risk of failure when posterior capsule is used for flap tissue, likely due to its tendency to curl rather than remain flat and fill the hole.

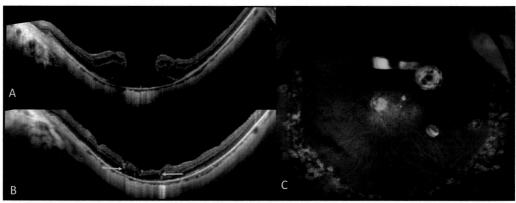

Figure 34-1. A persistent chronic macular hole (1100 μm) with retinal detachment following pars plana vitrectomy with ILM peel in a -15 diopter myope with a posterior staphyloma was closed using an autologous retinal free flap. (A) Preoperative OCT. (B) Postoperative OCT at month 3 with complete closure of the macular hole. The yellow arrows mark the edges of the retinal free flap. (C) Widefield color photo demonstrating the superotemporal harvest site.

Adjuvant Blood Products

Blood and blood components have both been used for some time in the closure of macular holes. These adjuvant blood products have included serum, platelet-rich plasma, and whole blood. These blood products are used after vitrectomy, with or without ILM peeling, during vitreous surgery. In the case of platelet-rich plasma, for example, blood is drawn from the patient and centrifuged to create a platelet-rich medium. The platelet concentrate is then mixed with a small amount of sodium chloride, and 2 or 3 drops are placed in the hole. Injection of autologous platelet concentrate has significantly improved anatomic success in patients with large macular holes.[6,7] The blood or platelet mixture acts as a plug to seal the hole, and growth factors within the blood components are thought to help with the proliferation of retinal tissue into the hole. Autologous blood has been used in combination with an ILM flap for myopic macular holes.[8]

Autologous Retinal Transplant (Retinal Free Flap)

The autologous retinal transplant for macular holes is a novel technique involving harvesting an autologous neurosensory retinal free flap from the retinal periphery and positioning it over the macular hole. Multiple hypotheses are involved in the mechanism of anatomical and functional improvement. This technique is used in refractory or recurrent cases when an ILM flap is not an option as the ILM has been previously peeled or in very large holes measuring more than 700 μm in diameter, even without prior ILM peeling. It was first described in and may be most useful in those patients with refractory myopic macular holes with associated foveoschisis or retinal detachment[9] (Figure 34-1).

Summary

A small group of macular holes—those that are large, chronic, or associated with high myopia, trauma, juxtafoveal telangiectasia, or retinal detachment—are often recalcitrant to closure with standard vitrectomy and ILM peeling. Vitreoretinal surgeons now have several evolving techniques to treat patients with chronic large macular holes. These techniques represent some of the newest innovations in vitreoretinal surgery to address challenging macular hole cases. These innovations have greatly improved anatomic and functional outcomes in patients with macular holes that would have been previously considered inoperable. It is important, however, to manage patient and referring provider expectations because in certain cases of chronic macular holes, hole closure may not be associated with significant visual improvement.

References

1. Bainbridge J, Herbert E, Gregor Z. Macular holes: vitreoretinal relationships and surgical approaches. *Eye.* 2008;22(10):1301-1309.
2. Fujikawa M, Kawamura H, Kakinoki M, et al. Scleral imbrication combined with vitrectomy and gas tamponade for refractory macular hole retinal detachment associated with high myopia. *Retina.* 2014;34(12):2451-2457.
3. Siam ALH, El Maamoun TA, Ali MH. Macular buckling for myopic macular hole retinal detachment. *Retina.* 2012;32(4):748-753.
4. Michalewska Z, Michalewski J, Adelman RA, Nawrocki J. Inverted internal limiting membrane flap technique for large macular holes. *Ophthalmology.* 2010;117(10):2018-2025.
5. Chen S-N, Yang C-M. Lens capsular flap transplantation in the management of refractory macular hole from multiple etiologies. *Retina.* 2016;36(1):163-170.
6. Paques M, Chastang C, Mathis A, et al; Platelets in Macular Hole Surgery Group. Effect of autologous platelet concentrate in surgery for idiopathic macular hole: results of a multicenter, double-masked, randomized trial. *Ophthalmology.* 1999;106(5):932-938.
7. Konstantinidis A, Hero M, Nanos P, Panos GD. Efficacy of autologous platelets in macular hole surgery. *Clin Ophthalmol.* 2013;7:745-750.
8. Lai C-C, Chen Y-P, Wang N-K, et al. Vitrectomy with internal limiting membrane repositioning and autologous blood for macular hole retinal detachment in highly myopic eyes. *Ophthalmology.* 2015;122(9):1889-1898.
9. Grewal DS, Mahmoud TH. Autologous neurosensory retinal free flap for closure of refractory myopic macular holes. *JAMA Ophthalmol.* 2016;134(2):229.

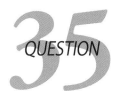

EXPLAIN ALL OF THESE NEW ANTICOAGULANTS TO ME. SHOULD I CONSIDER STOPPING THEM PREOPERATIVELY?

Elizabeth Verner-Cole, MD
Phoebe Lin, MD, PhD

Both thromboembolic and retinal disease occur more frequently in older patients and, with an increasing aging population, retinal surgeons will face a growing number of patients on anticoagulants. Given the complexities of retinal surgery, often involving highly vascular tissue, it is important to determine whether or not it is safe to proceed with surgery in patients on anticoagulants. Developed in 1954, Coumadin (warfarin) continues to be the most prescribed anticoagulant to date. Its method of action is via Vitamin K inhibition, ultimately decreasing levels of clotting factors X, IX, VII, and II (thrombin) as well as proteins C and S. Due to its indirect action on the clotting cascade as well as its many drug-drug and food-drug interactions, it can be difficult to obtain optimal anticoagulation. Studies show that up to 50% of the time, patients on warfarin are not within their target international normalized ratio (INR) range (typically INR = 2 to 3) and are thus either under- or over-coagulated.[1] For this reason, many new oral anticoagulants have been developed that inhibit a single factor in the coagulation cascade, providing a more direct and pharmacologically reliable effect. Initially labeled novel oral anticoagulants, they are also known as non–Vitamin K antagonist oral anticoagulants (NOACs) or direct oral anticoagulants (DOACs). The Food and Drug Administration–approved DOAC agents include the thrombin inhibitor Pradaxa (dabigatran) and the factor Xa inhibitors Xarelto (rivaroxaban), Eliquis (apixaban), and Savaysa (edoxaban) (Table 35-1). DOAC agents offer multiple advantages over warfarin, including fewer food and drug interactions, no need for repeated blood testing, rapid onset within 2 to 3 hours (compared to 2 to 3 days with warfarin), and lower risk of intracranial hemorrhage. Disadvantages of DOAC agents include limited ability to quickly reverse the anticoagulation effect (only dabigatran has an approved reversal agent, idarucizumab), altered metabolism in patients with renal insufficiency or over 75 years old, and increased risk of gastrointestinal bleeding.[2]

Fekrat S, ed. *Curbside Consultation in Retina: 49 Clinical Questions, Second Edition.* (pp 177-183).
© 2019 SLACK Incorporated

Table 35-1

Pharmacokinetics of Direct Oral Anticoagulant Agents

Drug	Target	Half-Life	Timing of Cessation for Low Bleed Risk Surgery	Timing of Cessation for High Bleed Risk Surgery
Dabigatran	Factor IIa	12 to 17 hours	≥24 hours before surgery	Last dose 4 to 5 days before surgery (depending on CrCl)
Rivaroxaban	Factor Xa	5 to 9 hours in healthy; 11 to 13 hours in elderly	≥24 hours before surgery	Last dose 3 days before surgery
Apixaban	Factor Xa	8 to 15 hours	≥24 hours before surgery	Last dose 3 days before surgery
Edoxaban	Factor Xa	10 to 14 hours	≥24 hours before surgery	Last dose 3 days before surgery

CrCl = creatinine clearance

Adapted from Dubois V, Dincq AS, Douxfils J, et al. Perioperative management of patients on direct oral anticoagulants. *Thromb J.* 2017;15:14.

Ocular Complications Associated
With Direct Oral Anticoagulants

While the safety of anticoagulant use during cataract surgery is well-established, the risk of continuing anticoagulation at the time of retinal surgery has not been tested extensively, particularly with DOAC agents. Table 35-2 lists the studies to date of retinal surgery performed in patients on anticoagulants including the DOAC agents. The rate of visually significant postoperative hemorrhage (vitreous, retinal, or choroidal) across the majority of these studies ranges from 10% to 13%, with most cases occurring in proliferative diabetic retinopathy.[3-13] This is comparable to the rate of postoperative hemorrhage seen in patients not on anticoagulants undergoing vitrectomy for diabetic retinopathy. In fact, 2 studies that were conducted to compare rates of vitreous hemorrhage after vitrectomy for diabetic retinopathy with and without bevacizumab showed a rate of recurrent vitreous hemorrhage as high as 27% without the use of preoperative bevacizumab.[14,15] The latter studies, however, did not control for patients on anticoagulation.

Shieh and colleagues[16] investigated overall ocular complications occurring in patients anticoagulated with DOACs, including patients who had complications associated with ocular surgery and patients who had not received recent ocular surgery. They reported one spontaneous submacular hemorrhage in a patient on apixiban with intermediate non-neovascular age-related macular degeneration. They also reported 2 patients on dabigatran, one of whom developed multiple recurrences of hyphema after Ahmed tube surgery for neovascular glaucoma in the setting of an ischemic retinal vein occlusion until switching to warfarin, after which the hyphema resolved. Despite a second patient stopping dabigatran 72 hours before surgery, he developed a hyphema and vitreous hemorrhage after pars plana vitrectomy, removal of an intraocular lens implant with placement of an anterior chamber lens, and this cleared on discontinuation of this DOAC, but then he had recurrent intraocular hemorrhage after restarting dabigatran. A repeat vitrectomy was necessary, and dabigatran was stopped, without further ocular complication. Shieh et al also reported 3 patients on rivaroxaban, one of whom had a spontaneous rhegmatogenous retinal detachment with massive subretinal hemorrhage and vitreous hemorrhage and who was switched to warfarin after repair without further complication. A second patient on rivaroxaban developed a spontaneous vitreous hemorrhage that resolved on its own and was not associated with retinal breaks or other retinal pathology. A third patient on rivaroxaban developed massive hemorrhagic conjunctival chemosis, hyphema, and vitreous hemorrhage, as well as hemorrhage of the eyelids and cheek after vitrectomy surgery to remove a lens fragment even though a subtenon rather than retrobulbar block was used.[16] In large non-inferiority trials comparing dabigatran to warfarin, ocular hemorrhage occurred but was considered minor and not vision-threatening.[17,18] However, there exists one case report of bilateral spontaneous choroidal hemorrhage, vitreous hemorrhage, and hyphema occurring with this agent.[19] Phase III clinical trials for the other DOAC agents have not reported consistent ocular complications.[20,21] The authors have an unpublished case of a postoperative suprachoroidal hemorrhage and hyphema occurring in a patient on apixiban who required a vitrectomy for a dislocated iris-sutured intraocular lens implant, who did not have this complication with 2 prior vitrectomies 10 years earlier, when she was on warfarin instead. A recent meta-analysis comparing DOACs and traditional anti-thrombotic drugs for bleeding complications found no significant difference in intraocular bleeding complications.[22]

Table 35-2

Studies Investigating Anticoagulation in Vitreoretinal Surgery

Study	*Anticoagulant or Antiplatelet Drug*	*Number of Cases (% Complications)*	*Complications*
Gainey et al (1989)[7]	Warfarin	6 (0)	None
McCormack et al (1993)[11]	Warfarin and nicoumalone	8 (0)	None
Narendran & Williamson (2003)[12]	Warfarin	7 (29)	1 choroidal detachment 1 recurrent VH
Dayani & Grand (2006)[5]	Warfarin	19 (11)	2 postoperative hemorrhage
Fu et al (2007)[6]	Warfarin	10 (10)	1 hemorrhage from scleral buckle external drainage
Brown & Mahmoud (2011)[3]	ASA, clopidogrel, warfarin	27 (11)	3 postoperative VH (1 reoperative)
Chandra et al (2011)[4]	Warfarin	60 (0)	No difference in complications between warfarin and control
Mason et al (2011)[10]	Warfarin	64 (1.6)	1 transient VH
	Clopidogrel	136 (3.7)	5 transient VH
Malik et al (2012)[9]	ASA, clopidogrel, warfarin	56 (13)	7 postoperative VH (4 reoperative)
Passemard et al (2012)[13]	Warfarin or similar ASA or clopidogrel	0 (0) 44 (20)	0 6 VH, 3 retinal hemorrhage
Grand & Walia (2016)[8]	DOAC agents	36 (11)	4 postoperative VH (2 reoperative)

ASA = aspirin; VH = vitreous hemorrhage

In summary, even though anecdotes and case series suggest that either spontaneous or postoperative intraocular bleeding complications with DOACs may exceed usual expectations in terms of severity or recurrence, larger studies looking at overall bleeding complications appear to show no significant difference with classic anticoagulants. The larger studies, however, were not designed to assess ocular complications. Furthermore, even though the studies in retinal surgery outlined in Table 35-2 are limited by their retrospective nature, small sample sizes, and limited discussion of intraoperative findings, they do provide evidence that retinal surgery with anticoagulation on board, even with the DOAC agents, likely poses no significant additional harm.

Perioperative Management of Patients on Direct Oral Anticoagulants

With increasing use of DOACs due to the advantages in ease of use and lower risk of certain bleeding complications compared with the classic vitamin K antagonists, it is important for surgeons to understand how to manage these agents perioperatively. This requires an assessment of thromboembolic risk while off anticoagulation vs the risk of visually significant bleeding while remaining on such a drug. In this regard, there is no algorithmic approach; an understanding of the patient's anatomy, surgical risk, and systemic risk, all of which are not very different than in patients on classic anticoagulants, is required. Discussion of these assessments with the DOAC-prescribing physician is of paramount importance and might be part of a checklist during the preoperative evaluation of the patient. With current small-gauge vitrectomy surgery techniques and even in typical scleral buckling surgery, minimal risk for bleeding occurs given the use of small incisions, and the decreased chance of hypotony during these procedures with the use of valved cannulas. However, in more complex cases, for instance, requiring the enlargement of a wound, or in a patient with a history of intra- or postoperative hemorrhagic ocular complications, one might consider cessation of these drugs. In the latter scenario, a discussion with the primary care doctor or cardiologist who prescribed the DOAC or classic anticoagulant should include an assessment of the patient's systemic risk. In general, a CHADS$_2$ (congestive heart failure; hypertension; age of 75 years or older; diabetes mellitus; prior stroke, transient ischemic attack, or thromboembolism) score of less than 5 with a history of prior thromboembolism during temporary interruption of anticoagulants, patients with atrial fibrillation and a prior stroke or transient ischemic attack occurring greater than 3 months before surgery, and any patient with a recent history of stroke or transient ischemic attack, are considered at high thromboembolic risk.[23] Timing of cessation depends on the DOAC agent that is being used, the risk for bleed during the surgery (for which there are no guidelines in terms of the various kinds of vitreoretinal surgery), the half-life of the drug, and systemic factors (see Table 35-1).

In the event of intraoperative hemorrhage, current surgical techniques typically allow for rapid cessation of bleeding by briefly raising the intraocular pressure (≥ 60 mmHg) or careful use of endocautery. Given the small but real risk of developing a thromboembolic event with perioperative cessation of anticoagulation,[24] most surgeons feel the benefits outweigh the risk when continuing anticoagulants at the time of surgery.

For patients on warfarin, there is no established limit as to the maximum INR allowed for retinal surgery. Based on informal polls and discussions among retinal surgeons, it seems most surgeons are comfortable operating at an INR of 3 or less. The general consensus is to check the INR the morning of surgery, or at least within 2 days prior to surgery. If the patient is on a DOAC agent or there are other health concerns, then it is important to discuss this with the patient's primary care provider prior to surgery to ensure there are no issues with their anticoagulant.

References

1. Sudharsan R, Simone KM, Anderson NP, Aguirre GD, Beltran WA. Acute and protracted cell death in light-induced retinal degeneration in the canine model of rhodopsin autosomal dominant retinitis pigmentosa. *Invest Ophthalmol Vis Sci.* 2017;58(1):270-281. doi: 10.1167/iovs.16-20749

2. Berson EL. Long-term visual prognoses in patients with retinitis pigmentosa: the Ludwig von Sallmann lecture. *Exp Eye Res.* 2007;85(1):7-14.

3. Retinal Information Network. http://www.sph.uth.tmc.edu/Retnet/. Accessed April 27, 2018.

4. Kiser AK, Dagnelie G. Reported effects of non-traditional treatments and complementary and alternative medicine by retinitis pigmentosa patients. *Clin Exp Optom.* 2008;91(2):166-76. doi: 10.1111/j.1444-0938.2007.00224.x

5. Berson EL, Rosner B, Sandberg MA, et al. A randomized trial of vitamin A and vitamin E supplementation for retinitis pigmentosa. *Arch Ophthalmol.* 1993;111(6):761-72.

6. Hoffman DR, Hughbanks-Wheaton DK, Spencer R, et al. Docosahexaenoic acid slows visual field progression in X-linked retinitis pigmentosa: ancillary outcomes of the DHAX trial. *Invest Ophthalmol Vis Sci.* 2015;56(11):6646-53. doi: 10.1167/iovs.15-17786

7. Pan ZH, Lu Q, Bi A, Dizhoor AM, Abrams GW. Optogenetic approaches to restoring vision. *Annu Rev Vis Sci.* 2015;1:185-210. doi: 10.1146/annurev-vision-082114-035532

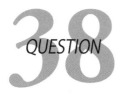

QUESTION

WHY SHOULD I SEND MY RETINAL DEGENERATION PATIENTS TO SPECIALISTS IF THERE IS NO CURE FOR THEIR CONDITION?

Alessandro Iannaccone, MD, MS, FARVO

There are a number of reasons why a retinal degeneration patient should be referred to a retinal degeneration specialist even if there is no fully-effective treatment or cure yet for these conditions.

One of the most important reasons is that reaching an accurate clinical and molecular genetic diagnosis is key. Retinal degenerations are a large group of heterogeneous conditions sharing features of progressive retinal degenerative damage that can be grossly differentiated in 2 subgroups: inherited (IRDs) and non-inherited ones. Typical IRDs include retinitis pigmentosa (RP), Leber congenital amaurosis, cone and cone-rod dystrophies, and related conditions, including complex syndromic ones and disorders that, while genetically affecting the entire retina, tend to affect clinically much more so the macular region, such as Stargardt disease (STGD), Best disease, macular pattern dystrophies and related entities.

Non-inherited retinal degenerations mainly include autoimmune retinopathies of the secondary paraneoplastic type (cancer-associated retinopathy [CAR]) or primary non-paraneoplastic type (AIR). CAR is the best-known one, but primary AIR is actually far more common. It is not uncommon that patients referred as suspected cases of simplex (isolated) RP do not actually have RP, but in fact AIR. Other clinical pictures mimicking IRDs develop in the broader family of AIR as well; thus, distinguishing true IRDs from AIR and CAR is very important not only to make the correct diagnosis but also because AIR and CAR are at least partially treatable, and there are very important systemic prognostic implications if a patient has CAR instead of RP.[1,2] This differential diagnostic task can be particularly challenging when a patient does not have a history of neoplastic disease.

Fekrat S, ed. *Curbside Consultation in Retina: 49 Clinical Questions, Second Edition.* (pp 197-201).
© 2019 SLACK Incorporated

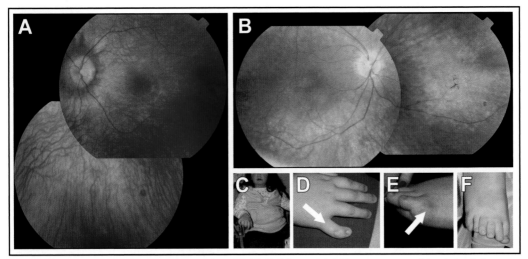

Figure 38-1. Spectrum of presentation in the BBS. (A) Children with BBS can present with minimal changes, limited to mild vascular attenuation to (B) more overtly degenerative phenotypes with marked vascular attenuation, waxy disc pallor, and a generalized dystrophic appearance of the retina with initial bone spicule-like deposits. Note also the macular retinal pigment epithelium drop-out and the loss of foveal reflex in B, which is a typical presentation for BBS. These patients may appear to have a fair preservation of the ellipsoid zone on optical coherence tomography, but it is usually very faint, as common in ciliopathies, and associated with signal loss on autofluorescence. Systemic characteristics of BBS include (C) early-onset obesity, (D) clynodactyly of the fifth finger with scars from removed extra appendages of either fingers or (E) toes, up to (F) full-fledged polydactyly. Syndactyly or brachydactyly can also be observed in BBS.

Focusing on IRDs, reaching a precise clinical and molecular genetic diagnosis has very important counseling, prognostic and, in some cases, current or immediately forthcoming treatment implications. From a clinical standpoint, the differential diagnosis of IRDs can be challenging and very time consuming. Many times, you need to ask numerous targeted systemic questions, which normal review of systems questionnaires do not cover, to recognize that an RP patient does not have just RP but may have hearing loss because of Usher syndrome or Refsum disease, or that a patient seemingly affected with Leber congenital amaurosis is in fact at risk for kidney failure from having instead the Senior-Loken syndrome or the Bardet-Biedl syndrome (BBS), and so on. Examples of some of these more complex and challenging presentations are illustrated in Figures 38-1 and 38-2. A referral to a retinal degeneration specialist, who has also this broader expertise and is comfortable with all these nuances of IRD-related syndromes and the ophthalmic genetic underpinnings thereof will give you the peace of mind of knowing that these subtler, but very important, aspects will not be missed.

Establishing the inheritance pattern of an IRD is also a top priority from a counseling perspective. A retinal degeneration specialist will take care of this for you, and your patient will not need to go see a medical geneticist for further counseling. The latter is an extra expense for your patient, more time spent away from work engaging in clinical care, and it will not always be effective if the medical geneticist is not familiar with the specific IRD affecting your patient. The optimal setting is when the retinal degeneration specialist works in tandem with a genetic counselor who can assist with the collection of the family trees, coordinate the molecular genetic diagnostic testing and the counseling both at the time of the visit and subsequently, when molecular genetic test results become available. Take the example of a simplex male RP patient. Let's assume he meets all the diagnostic criteria for RP. A common question you will be asked is, "What are the odds of my children becoming affected with RP?" When there is a family history of RP the counseling is easier, but when history is lacking, the most likely genetic inheritance pattern is autosomal

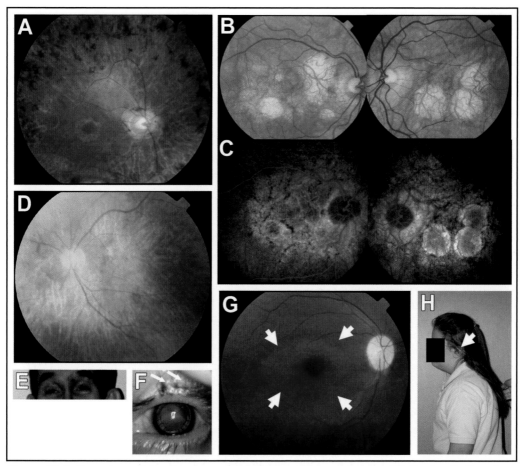

Figure 38-2. Sensorineural hearing loss retinal degeneration syndromes. (A) Fundus findings in a 56-year-old patient with Usher syndrome Type IIA (USH2A), exhibiting typical RP with marked vascular attenuation and diffuse bone spicule-like deposits, symmetrically distributed between the 2 eyes. In USH2A, a Bull's eye maculopathy is also often observed, as in the case presented here. The hearing loss of USH2A is congenital, affecting mainly the high frequencies and causing a typical wisp in the patient's speech. Night blindness is the rule in Usher syndrome. Other conditions present with post-verbal hearing loss, which does not compromise speech. One such example is Refsum disease. (B) Here we see the macular region of a 49-year-old woman with blurred vision, photophobia, a geographic atrophy-like clinical phenotype, and a 5-year history of insulin-dependent diabetes. (C) The angiogram reveals a streaky pattern of fine pigmentary changes typical for an advanced stage of a macular pattern dystrophy, as seen in the mitochondrial disease known as the *maternally-inherited diabetes mellitus and deafness* syndrome. About 2% of diabetics are estimated to have maternally-inherited diabetes mellitus and deafness. (D) Peripapillary and posterior pole retinal pigment epithelium and retinal atrophy and (E, F) bilateral ptosis in the context of progressive chronic external ophthalmoplegia characterize the cone-rod dystrophy of another mitochondrial disease, Kearns-Sayre syndrome (KSS). All manifestations in KSS are highly variable, and hearing loss can range from complete and congenital (like in Usher syndrome Type I) to mild and postverbal. This patient also required a penetrating keratoplasty to manage the rare finding of (F) marked corneal clouding, and (E, arrows in F) a blepharoplasty. Another key feature of KSS is predisposition to sudden heart block, requiring prophylactic pacemaker implantation. (G) An oval area of bull's eye–like macular discoloration (arrows) and temporal pallor characterize the cone-rod dystrophy of Alström syndrome (ALMS), an obesity-hearing loss syndrome (H, and arrows pointing to a hearing aid device) with features overlapping also with BBS. Hearing loss is usually postverbal. Infantile-onset dilated cardiomyopathy is classic for ALMS. Unlike BBS, abnormal extremities are absent in ALMS.

recessive, but studies have shown that about 16% of these patients actually have X-linked RP,[3] and a *de novo* dominant mutation, however rare an event, cannot be excluded either. A dedicated work-up by retinal degeneration specialists and their team will ensure that your patient receives adequate counseling from this perspective, proper molecular genetic diagnostic testing, and subsequently proper explanation of any and all findings.

Another challenge that retinal degeneration specialists and their teams can best handle for you and for your patients is the interpretation of the far-from-uncommon novel mutations or genetic variants of unknown significance.[4] This issue has been a long-standing concern with highly polymorphic genes like the *ABCA4* gene that is responsible for STGD and other related conditions, and is becoming an increasingly prevalent problem with broad next generation sequencing diagnostic panels offered by a variety of laboratories. The challenge of relaying these results to patients and placing them into proper context is something that retinal degeneration specialists and their teams can handle far better for your patients with IRDs.

Another very frequent question that IRD patients will ask you is, "How much time will it take before I go blind"? Most IRDs do not cause complete blindness, but usually progress *only* to legal blindness by either visual field or visual acuity criteria (or both). Once an inheritance pattern is clearly identified, the disease-causing gene is discovered, and the disease-causing mutations are identified, specialists in retinal degenerations and their team will be in the best position to relay to your patient the significance of the identified genetic changes from a prognostic point of view. The natural history of IRDs is incompletely understood in many cases, and significant systematic multicenter efforts are underway to fill this gap for a number of conditions (eg, the ProgStar study for STGD).[5,6] Similar efforts, supported by federal and foundation grants as well as by various companies, are ongoing for certain forms of dominant and X-linked RP, achromatopsia, USH2A, and choroideremia. Understanding well the natural history of each IRD is essential not only to give your patients answers to the, "How much time will it take before I go blind" question, but is critical to identifying adequate outcome measures for clinical trials. Retinal degeneration specialists are either intimately aware of the results of the published studies or, in fact, are actively participating in them. In addition, many of these natural history studies are being conducted in parallel to Phase I gene therapy trials (or other interventional studies) or are directly leading up to them, and many retinal degeneration specialists are involved with these trials as well. Thus, a referral to a retinal degeneration specialist may not only help getting your patient enrolled in one of these natural history studies, which will inform us all better about the natural history of these specific conditions, but is likely to open a direct door to treatment for your patients or one of their affected family members.

Referring your IRD patients to a retinal degeneration specialist will help also from a therapeutic perspective. While no cures for most IRDs exist yet, some treatments, albeit capable only of slowing disease progression and despite some controversy about them, actually exist for IRDs. Examples of these include the vitamin A and the lutein supplementation trials of RP, which I have reviewed elsewhere.[7] You need to know what dosing is appropriate for your patient and if such treatments are appropriate. A retinal degeneration specialist will also be far more up-to-date with the latest scientific developments in other nutrition-based and pharmacologic approaches that are under investigation, and will be able to counsel your IRD patients best with evidence-based information as to which of them may be most appropriate for their condition. In addition, there is now a US Food and Drug Administration–approved gene therapy available for the specific form of RP linked to the *RPE65* gene (Luxturna, Spark Therapeutics). Genetic testing is absolutely necessary to determine if a patient is eligible for treatment with this approach.

At times, you need to know what supplements your patient should not take to avoid hastening the progression of the disease. For example, unlike RP, in molecularly confirmed STGD due to *ABCA4* mutations, the current understanding is that use of vitamin A– or beta carotene–containing supplements could be harmful, so much so that treatment trials are underway to inhibit vitamin A delivery to the retina of STGD patients (NCT03033108) or to treat them with modified forms of vitamin A that, based on solid experimental data, should not lead to the accumulation of the expected toxic metabolites (NCT02402660). Thus, while these trials are yet to be completed, there is a solid rationale to at least advise STGD patients to avoid Vitamin A– or beta carotene–containing supplements. The genetic testing for *ABCA4* disease-causing changes can address this issue as well. The same applies to vitamin E supplements for RP.[7] You would not believe how many RP or STGD patients are incorrectly counseled to take regular multivitamins, which invariably contain large amounts of such potentially harmful supplements, or even supplements that may be appropriate for age-related macular degeneration, but not for RP or STGD.

Finally, some common complications in RP and related disorders are treatable too. One perfect example is cystoid macular edema (CME).[7] The CME of RP is not the same as the CME of Irvine-Gass syndrome, which is driven by perioperative inflammation in the anterior segment, and benefits from treatments such as oral and/or topical carbonic anhydrase inhibitors or posteriorly delivered (periocular or intravitreal) steroids.[7] A retinal degeneration specialist is going to be intimately aware of all these subtleties in the recommendations that can be made to your IRD patient and will be able to provide detailed input of therapeutic relevance to your patient precisely and effortlessly.

References

1. Heckenlively JR, Ferreyra HA. Autoimmune retinopathy: a review and summary. *Semin Immunopathol.* 2008;30:127-134.
2. Ferreyra HA, Jayasundera T, Khan NW, He S, Lu Y, Heckenlively JR. Management of autoimmune retinopathies with immunosuppression. *Arch Ophthalmol.* 2009;127:390-397.
3. Branham K, Othman M, Brumm M, et al. Mutations in RPGR and RP2 account for 15% of males with simplex retinal degenerative disease. *Invest Ophthalmol Vis Sci.* 2012;53:8232-8237.
4. Chan SC, MacDonald IM. Resolving genetic test results for the patient and the clinician. *Am J Ophthalmol.* 2016;170:xiv-xvi.
5. Kong X, Strauss RW, Michaelides M, et al. Visual acuity loss and associated risk factors in the Retrospective Progression of Stargardt Disease Study (ProgStar Report No. 2). *Ophthalmology.* 2016;123:1887-1897.
6. Strauss RW, Ho A, Munoz B, et al. The Natural History of the Progression of Atrophy Secondary to Stargardt Disease (ProgStar) Studies: design and baseline characteristics: progstar report no. 1. *Ophthalmology.* 2016;123:817-828.
7. Iannaccone A, Berdia J. Retinitis Pigmentosa. Review No. 21. Danbury, CT: National Organization for Rare Disorders, Inc. https://www.researchgate.net/publication/320557157_Retinitis_Pigmentosa. Published 2012. Retrieved May 29, 2018.

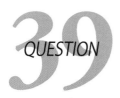

WHAT IS THE ARTIFICIAL RETINAL PROSTHESIS (ARGUS II IMPLANT) AND WHO WOULD BE A GOOD CANDIDATE FOR IT?

Paul Hahn, MD, PhD

The Argus II retinal prosthesis is an implant designed to restore visual stimulation previously considered permanently lost. It is the only retinal prosthesis currently approved by the US Food and Drug Administration (FDA; 2013). It has additionally received the Conformité Européenne (CE; 2011) mark and has been approved by Health Canada (2015). The Argus II includes an external (wearable) and internal (surgically implanted) component. The external equipment consists of glasses, a video processing unit (VPU), and a wired cable (Figure 39-1A). The glasses hold a video micro-camera in the nasal bridge that transmits images to the wired VPU for image processing. The VPU transforms the images to data that are then transmitted wirelessly to the internal implant in the eye, which also receives power wirelessly via induction from the external hardware.

The implanted component consists of a receiving coil and electronics case secured to the eye in a scleral buckle fashion and a 60-electrode array secured to the inner surface of the retina with a retinal tack (Figure 39-1B). The data sent from the external VPU wirelessly to the implanted electronics package stimulates the array to emit small pulses of electricity that excite remaining viable inner retina cells, including ganglion cells. These artificially stimulated retinal ganglion cells transmit signals through their axons to the lateral geniculate nucleus and then the occipital cortex, which perceives patterns of light. The final step is for patients to piece together these patterns of light to form vision.[1]

When I evaluate a patient interested in this technology, I first confirm that they fit the approved indications. The Argus II is currently FDA-approved for a defined subset of patients: adults (age 25 years or older) with a diagnosis of retinitis pigmentosa (RP) and a history of prior useful vision who have progressed to bare or no light perception vision in both eyes. Although I tell patients

Fekrat S, ed. *Curbside Consultation in Retina: 49 Clinical Questions, Second Edition.* (pp 203-205).
© 2019 SLACK Incorporated

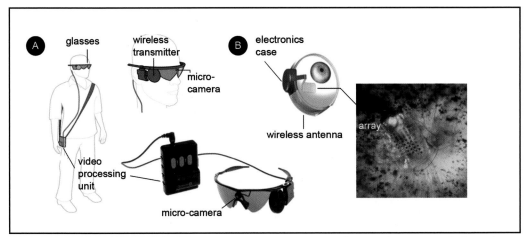

Figure 39-1. Argus II retinal prosthesis components. (A) Diagram of external portion including glasses with micro-camera, wireless transmitter (radio frequency coil), and VPU (Reprinted with permission from Second Sight Medical Products, Inc.). (B) Diagram of the surgically implanted component including the electronics case, the wireless antenna, and the 60-electrode array (Reprinted with permission from Second Sight Medical Products, Inc.) with photograph identifying an Argus array optimally centered on the macula and attached to the retina by a retinal tack (image courtesy of Paul Hahn, MD, PhD).

that other diseases may also benefit from the Argus II, the only on-label indication is currently for end-stage RP. Contraindications include comorbidities that would prevent the implant from functioning properly (eg, optic nerve disease, cortical blindness, prior retinal detachment, retinal vascular occlusion, trauma, and severe strabismus). Other contraindications include conditions that would prevent adequate implantation of the Argus II, such as conjunctival thinning, axial length less than 20.5 mm or greater than 26 mm (given the fixed intraocular cable length), and conditions that prevent implant visualization, such as corneal opacities. Phakic patients will also require removal of the lens prior to or during Argus II implantation. Finally, the implant is not recommended in patients with a tendency to eye rubbing or with a metallic or active implantable device in the head, such as a cochlear implant.

Beyond these eligibility criteria, I utilize my initial evaluation with patients to determine if they view this novel technology with the appropriate perspective, which I feel is one of the most important criteria in selecting an ideal candidate. As with any prosthesis, the Argus II requires significant rehabilitation to maximize its utility. I explain that after a 3- to 5-hour surgery and a standard postoperative recovery, the device will be programmed over the course of several days and then turned on for the first time a few weeks after surgery. Although patients will start to experience flashes of lights immediately at the time the device is first turned on, I emphasize that they will likely not be able to interpret these flashes early on. Rather, the patient will undergo months of low vision rehabilitation and occupational therapy to teach him or her how to use the device and maximize its utility in his or her own environment. Beyond these few months, each patient should look forward to a lifelong journey as he or she becomes increasingly familiar with this new visual stimulation. Many patients may expect a "plug-and-play" device with minimal effort from their part, and I discourage such patients from the early generation of this technology.

Patients want to know what they will see with this device. I inform them up front that they will not be able to read, drive, or even recognize faces, which are often what patients would most like to recover. For those not immediately discouraged, I explain that the Argus II provides a new type of visual stimulation that is different than what normally sighted people see. It provides flashes of light that can allow patients to localize objects and identify movements.[1,2] Patients report being able to determine where surrounding people are standing, which improves their sense of social connectedness, one of the most important benefits of this device. They may be able to localize their dinner plate or a glass of water; follow the straight lines of a crosswalk; "see" the location of a loved one's face; and identify doorways and windows. Although in isolation, many of these percepts may be difficult to interpret, Argus II users learn to place these visual stimuli in context in conjunction with stimuli from their other senses to provide another dimension to orient themselves. Many patients with chronic end-stage vision loss have adapted well and may be looking for more than this device can offer. However, certain pioneering patients may be excited by the possibility of exploring another dimension of visual stimulation to replace the traditional vision they had lost. When I meet these latter patients with profound vision loss from end-stage RP, I am excited to be able offer the Argus II as an option. To me, these are the ideal candidates.[3]

I often evaluate patients with vision loss from disease conditions other than RP. Although I explain they do not currently fit the on-label indication, I encourage them that the Argus II heralds the onset of a thrilling era of regenerative and restorative medicine. The Argus II has only been formally evaluated in patients with RP, but a pilot study evaluating its use in advanced dry age-related macular degeneration is currently underway; similarly, this device may prove to benefit other retinal degenerations as well. Beyond the Argus II, another retinal prosthesis—the Alpha IMS, a light-sensitive subretinal implant—has received the European CE mark in 2013 for end-stage RP patients. More recently in 2016, the Pixium Vision Iris II, a 150-electrode epiretinal implant, received the CE mark for outer retinal degenerations. These implants provide other options for some patients, but there have not yet been any comparative studies across these platforms. Other retinal implants are still in development or clinical trials.[4] There are also several alternative implant-based approaches in early phases of development that aim to restore vision. These include cortical prostheses that directly stimulate the occipital cortex, neurotransmitter based retinal prostheses, and photovoltaic cellular approaches. In addition, there are sensory substitution devices, such as auditory, tactile, and tongue-stimulating devices.

Although the technology is early, the Argus II marks an exciting era of enthusiasm and hope for physicians and patients in the treatment of vision previously considered permanently lost. This device represents the first approved device to artificially stimulate the retina and restore vision. Although still far from natural vision, and although currently only approved for patients with profound vision loss from RP, retinal implants and their early successes encourage development of future technologies towards improved safety, durability, and image resolution with the hope of restored vision for all blindness.

References

1. Ho AC, Humayun MS, Dorn JD, et al. Long-term results from an epiretinal prosthesis to restore sight to the blind. *Ophthalmology*. 2015;122(8):1547–1554.
2. Dorn JD, Ahuja AK, Caspi A, et al. The detection of motion by blind subjects with the epiretinal 60-electrode (Argus II) retinal prosthesis. *JAMA Ophthalmol*. 2013;131(2):183-189.
3. Ghodasra DH, Chen A, Arevalo JF, et al. Worldwide Argus II implantation: recommendations to optimize patient outcomes. *BMC Ophthalmol*. 2016;16:52.
4. Chapter 1—restoring vision to the blind: the new age of implanted visual prostheses. *Trans Vis Sci Technol*. 2014;3(7):3. doi: 10.1167/tvst.3.7.3

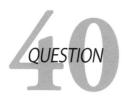

QUESTION

HOW DO YOU DIFFERENTIATE BETWEEN RETINOSCHISIS AND RETINAL DETACHMENT?

Scott Ketner, MD

Ron A. Adelman, MD, MPH, MBA, FARVO

Retinoschisis is a splitting of the retinal layers, most often at the outer plexiform layer or the nerve fiber layer.[1-3] By contrast, a retinal detachment is a separation of the neurosensory retina from the retinal pigment epithelium (RPE).

Peripheral, degenerative retinoschisis is thought to develop with the coalescence of cystic lesions in areas of peripheral cystoid degeneration, as the degeneration of neuroretinal and glial supporting elements allows a splitting to occur within the retinal layers. The newly created space fills with a mucopolysaccharide substance.[1-3] By contrast, a retinal detachment (ie, a rhegmatogenous retinal detachment [RRD]) develops when fluid from the vitreous cavity gains access, via a retinal break, to the potential space between the neurosensory retina and RPE.

Retinoschisis rarely progresses posteriorly to encroach on the macula and can usually be observed. Attempts to treat schisis with laser barricade to prevent posterior progression are likely to be ineffective and can expose the patient to unnecessary risks.[4-7] A RRD, by contrast, almost always progresses if left treated. In rare cases, in which both an inner and outer retinal hole develop within an area of schisis, a schisis can cause a retinal detachment; fortunately, this is rare.[4]

Peripheral retinoschisis can resemble a RRD. Both can appear as elevated peripheral lesions; however, the following characteristics can help differentiate the 2 (Table 40-1).

Fekrat S, ed. *Curbside Consultation in Retina: 49 Clinical Questions, Second Edition.* (pp 207-210).
© 2019 SLACK Incorporated

Table 40-1
Summarizing Distinguishing Features of Retinoschisis and Retinal Detachment

	Retinoschisis	*Retinal Detachment*
Location	Often inferotemporal, frequently bilateral	Not as strongly associated with a particular quadrant or with bilaterality
Appearance	More diaphanous, thinner, more transparent, more dome-shaped, with fewer surface wrinkles	Less diaphanous, less dome-shaped, with more surface wrinkles
Response to scleral depression	Tends not to flatten with scleral depression	Tends to partially flatten with scleral depression
Humphrey Visual Field Defect	Absolute	Relative
T-sign	T-shaped shadow not seen by patient	T-shaped shadow seen by patient
OCT	Shows splitting within the neurosensory retina—NFL or OPL	Shows separation between the RPE and neurosensory retina
Laser photocoagulation	Laser tends not to "take"	Laser does tend to "take"

NFL = nerve fiber layer; OPL = outer plexiform layer; OCT = optical coherence tomography

Location

Schisis most often occurs in the inferotemporal periphery and is frequently bilateral.[4,5]

Appearance on Indirect Ophthalmoscopy

Compared to a retinal detachment, a schisis tends to be appear more diaphanous, more dome-shaped, less mobile, and to have less surface wrinkling.

Response to Scleral Depression

Scleral depression tends to partially flatten a retinal detachment, as the subretinal fluid is pushed through the retinal break into the vitreous cavity, whereas a schisis is unlikely to flatten with depression because the fluid tends to be trapped within the schisis cavity.

Visual Field Testing

A schisis will produce an absolute visual field defect because the connections between the inner and outer retina have been severed. By contrast, a retinal detachment will tend to produce only a relative field defect, as the neurosensory retina is still essentially intact, though separated from the underlying RPE and choroidal blood supply.

T-Sign on Indirect Ophthalmoscopy Perimetry

When held on the observer's side of the condensing lens during indirect ophthalmoscopy, a Schocket scleral depressor can be used to project a T-shaped shadow onto the area of interest (schisis or detachment). Patients with a detachment will be able to appreciate the T-shaped shadow (T-sign), whereas patients with a schisis will not, as their scotoma is absolute.[8]

Optical Coherence Tomography

It is not always possible to obtain OCT images of the peripheral lesion in question, but when able to be obtained, OCT images can show whether there is a split within the neurosensory retina (in the case of a schisis) or between the retina and the RPE (in the case of a detachment).[9]

Laser Photocoagulation

When applied to a schisis, argon laser will tend to cause a visible whitening of the outer retina, as the energy absorbed by the RPE cells generates edema in the overlying outer retinal cells.[10] By contrast, laser tends not to produce whitening when applied to a detachment because the RPE cells capable of absorbing the laser energy are separated from the detached retina by subretinal fluid. However, it should be noted that some authors question the utility of this test, noting that retinal whitening can sometimes be achieved in areas with overlying detached retina, especially if the laser power is turned high enough.[9,11]

References

1. Lewis H. Peripheral retinal degenerations and the risk of retinal detachment. *Am J Ophthalmol*. 2003;136(1):155-160.
2. Straatsma BR, Foos RY. Typical and reticular degenerative retinoschisis. *Am J Ophthalmol*. 1973;75:551.
3. Zimmerman LE, Spencer WH. The pathologic anatomy of retinoschisis. *AMA Arch Ophthalmol*. 1960;63(1):10-19.
4. Byer NE. Clinical study of senile retinoschisis. *Arch Ophthalmol*. 1968;79(1):36-44.
5. Buch H, Vinding T, Nielsen NV. Prevalence and long-term natural course of retinoschisis among elderly individuals: the Copenhagen City Eye Study. *Ophthalmology*. 2007;114(4):751-755.
6. Byer NE. The long-term natural history of senile retinoschisis with implications for management. *Ophthalmology*. 1986;93:1127.
7. Byer NE. Perspectives on the management of the complications of senile retinoschisis. *Eye (Lond)*. 2002;16(4):359-364.
8. Kylstra JA, Holdren DN. Indirect ophthalmoscope perimetry in patients with retinal detachment or retinoschisis. *Am J Ophthalmol*. 1995;119(4):521-522.

9. Ip M, Garza-Karren C, Duker JS, et al. Differentiation of degenerative retinoschisis from retinal detachment using optical coherence tomography. *Ophthalmology*. 1999;106(3):600-605.

10. Okun E, Cibis PA. The role of photocoagulation in the management of retinoschisis. *Arch Ophthalmol*. 1964;72: 309–314.

11. Landers MB III, Robinson CH. Photocoagulation in the diagnosis of senile retinoschisis. *Am J Ophthalmol*. 1977;84:18–23.

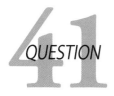

WHAT SYSTEMIC CONDITIONS ARE ASSOCIATED WITH AN INCREASED RISK OF RETINAL DETACHMENT? WHAT SHOULD I DO ABOUT IT?

Joseph N. Martel, MD
Mallika Doss, MD

The risk of rhegmatogenous retinal detachment (RRD) is increased in systemic diseases (Table 41-1) that fundamentally result in abnormal vitreous, atypical vitreoretinal traction, predisposing vitreoretinal lesions, or other anatomical ocular abnormalities. While there are systemic disorders associated with exudative retinal detachment (eg, eclampsia, Vogt-Koyanagi-Harada syndrome, metastasis, vascular malformations), the focus of this chapter will be on systemic conditions that increase the risk of RRD.

Inherent Vitreoretinal Abnormalities

Stickler syndrome (hereditary progressive arthro-ophthalmopathy) is perhaps the most important hereditary systemic disorder associated with RRD. This condition portends about a 50% lifetime risk of RRD. It is a connective tissue disorder caused by defect in Type II procollagen[1] and characterized as a hyaloideoretinopathy, whose hallmark is vitreous liquefaction (optically empty vitreous) and adherent cortical vitreous remnants behind the lens.[2] In addition to an anomalous vitreous, patients with Stickler syndrome often have ocular anatomical predispositions to retinal detachment, such as high axial myopia and perivascular radial lattice degeneration with strong vitreous adhesions along the borders of these lesions.[3] Retinal breaks are often numerous with variable distances from the vitreous base region.[4] Systemic findings in Stickler syndrome may include hearing impairment, arthritis, skeletal abnormalities, cleft palate, bifid uvula, and

Fekrat S, ed. *Curbside Consultation in Retina: 49 Clinical Questions, Second Edition.* (pp 211-213).
© 2019 SLACK Incorporated

Table 41-1

Systemic Conditions Associated With Rhegmatogenous Retinal Detachment

Inherent Vitreoretinal Abnormalities	• Stickler syndrome • Marfan syndrome • Ehlers-Danlos syndrome • Homocystinuria
Acquired Vitreoretinal Abnormalities	*Proliferative Retinopathies* • Diabetes mellitus • Sickling hemoglobinopathies • Hypertension *Infectious Uveitis* • Necrotizing herpetic retinitis *Traumatic/Self-induced* • Atopic dermatitis[4,5] • Cognitive disability

flattening of the mid-face.[4] Additionally, about 12% of patients with Pierre Robin sequence (cleft palate, micrognathia, and glossoptosis) suffer from Stickler syndrome.

Marfan syndrome, Ehlers-Danlos syndrome, and homocystinuria are all hereditary systemic connective tissue disorders which influence collagen cross-linking causing thin and collapsible sclera. The result is sclera that is less elastic and prone to stretching, resulting in axial myopia and crystalline lens subluxation. It is thought that vitreoretinal abnormalities associated with high myopia, accelerated vitreous degeneration, and subluxation of the crystalline lens influence the rate of RRD.[6] The association of lens dislocation and retinal detachment is likely from disruption of the normal barrier function of the crystalline lens and zonules resulting in accelerated vitreous liquefaction. Intraocular surgery to remove the dislocated crystalline lens secondarily increases the risk of retinal detachment and is associated with a higher incidence of vitreous loss.[4] Indeed, any systemic diseases or syndromes that result in high axial myopia consequently increase the risk of RRD because increased myopia is positively correlated with increasing incidence and severity of vitreous liquefaction. Predisposing retinal lesions, such as lattice degeneration, is common in these systemic diseases.

In all of these systemic connective tissue disorders, the inherent risk of RRD warrants close surveillance with scleral depressed fundus examination. Aggressive treatment of retinal breaks and prophylactic laser retinopexy treatment of lattice degeneration are advised. The need for multiple surgical repairs is common in these syndromic RRD cases and surgery is often more technically challenging than nonsyndromic RRD cases.[3]

Acquired Vitreoretinal Abnormalities

Proliferative retinopathy is the result of several systemic conditions, including diabetes mellitus, hypertension, sickling hemoglobinopathies, and other conditions causing retinal ischemia. While proliferative retinopathy most commonly causes tractional retinal detachments, RRDs can result secondarily.[2] Neovascular tufts on the retina create firm vitreoretinal adhesions. When these vessels regress, the contracting force creates excess traction on the ischemic and atrophic retina resulting in retinal breaks.

Similarly, infectious uveitic conditions, notably necrotizing herpetic retinitis, can secondarily cause atrophic retinal breaks resulting in RRD. Fifty percent of patients with necrotizing herpetic retinitis develop retinal detachments that frequently have multiple, large, or posterior retinal breaks and may also involve proliferative vitreoretinopathy.[4]

Self-induced trauma, such as excessive eye-rubbing, can increase a patient's risk for developing a retinal detachment. This external manipulation creates repetitive anterior-posterior vitreous traction.[4] Self-induced ocular trauma is often involuntary and seen in young patients with atopic dermatitis and patients with mental retardation.

Close surveillance with a dilated fundus examination with scleral depression for patients with acquired systemic conditions that predispose to retinal detachments is recommended. For patients with tractional or combined tractional/RRD in association with proliferative retinopathies, vitreoretinal surgery with panretinal photocoagulation is performed to cause regression of the retinal neovascularization and reattach the retina.[2]

Depending on the underlying systemic disease and the characteristics of any high-risk vitreoretinal lesions, prophylactic laser treatment, and even prophylactic scleral buckling, has been proposed in some high-risk patients.[7] Patients and their caretakers should be counseled about their lifelong risk of developing a retinal detachment and be aware of the hallmark symptoms (ie, flashes, floaters, visual field loss). Prompt referral to a vitreoretinal specialist is necessary in the event of a newly diagnosed retinal break or retinal detachment.

References

1. Ang A, Poulson AV, Goodburn SF, Richards AJ, Scott JD, Snead MO. Retinal detachment and prophylaxis in type 1 Stickler syndrome. *Ophthalmology*. 2008;115(1):164-168.
2. Schubert HD. 2013-2014 Basic and Clinical Science Course, Section 12: Retina and Vitreous. San Francisco, CA: American Academy of Ophthalmology.
3. Reddy DN, Yonekawa Y, Thomas BJ, Nudleman ED, William GA. Long-term surgical outcomes of retinal detachment in patients with Stickler Syndrome. *Clin Ophthalmol*. 2016;10:1531-1534.
4. Benson WE, Regillo CD. *Retinal Detachment: Diagnosis and Management*. 3rd ed. Lippincott-Raven, 1998.
5. Sasoh M, Mitzuani H, Matsubara H, et al. Incidence of retinal detachment associated with atopic dermatitis in Japan: a review of cases from 1992 to 2011. *Clin Ophthalmol*. 2015;9:1129-1134.
6. Lowenstein A, Barequet JS, De Juan E Jr, Maumenee IH. Retinal detachment in Marfan syndrome. *Retina*. 2000;20(4):358-363.
7. Freeman HM. Fellow eyes of non-traumatic giant retinal breaks. In: Ryan SJ, ed. *Retina*, 3rd ed. St. Louis, MO: Mosby; 2013: 1850.

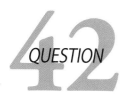

WHAT RETINAL FINDINGS SHOULD BE TREATED BEFORE CATARACT SURGERY, REFRACTIVE SURGERY, OR YTTRIUM-ALUMINUM-GARNET LASER?

Franco M. Recchia, MD

The goal of prophylactic retinal treatment is to reduce the chance of postsurgical complications related to vitreoretinal disorders. These potential complications include rhegmatogenous retinal detachment (RRD), macular edema, and progression of vision-threatening retinopathy.

RRD typically arises from vitreous traction on the peripheral retina leading to peripheral retinal breaks. Peripheral vitreoretinal traction often occurs in the setting of posterior vitreous detachment. Posterior vitreous detachment formation can be accelerated by anterior movement of the vitreous following cataract extraction or following yttrium-aluminum-garnet (YAG) laser capsulotomy.[1] It has been speculated that LASIK may also alter the vitreoretinal interface via compression/decompression changes in the anteroposterior axis induced during intraoperative suction. Retinal breaks are more likely to occur in areas of particularly adherent vitreous and/or retinal weakness.

Retinal or systemic conditions that may predispose to the development of a RRD include retinal break, lattice degeneration, vitreous hemorrhage, high myopia, RRD in the fellow eye, family history of RRD, premature birth, and systemic collagen disorders (specifically Stickler syndrome). Preoperative retinopexy with laser photocoagulation or cryotherapy should be applied to all symptomatic retinal breaks and all horseshoe retinal tears whether symptomatic or not. Retinopexy is strongly recommended to areas of lattice retinal degeneration in patients with a history of lattice-associated RRD in the fellow eye. Asymptomatic operculated holes and atrophic holes do not necessarily require treatment, but the option of treatment should be discussed with the patient. Prophylactic cryotherapy or *laser cerclage* (360° photocoagulation placed posterior to the vitreous base) is recommended in patients with genetic proof or high clinical suspicion of

Fekrat S, ed. *Curbside Consultation in Retina: 49 Clinical Questions, Second Edition.* (pp 215-218).
© 2019 SLACK Incorporated

Stickler syndrome. This hereditary disorder of connective tissue (caused by mutations in Type II collagen) is characterized by high myopia, early cataract, cleft palate, mid-facial flattening, hearing loss, cardiac and joint abnormalities, and strong family history of these symptoms and carries a risk of bilateral RRD approaching 75%.[2] Laser cerclage is also advisable in cases of high myopia (especially > 15 diopters) and in eyes of patients with poor visual acuity in the fellow eye, particularly for patients in whom postoperative follow-up or cooperation is limited.

Given the strong association (up to 70%) of peripheral retinal breaks in nondiabetic eyes with vitreous hemorrhage, these eyes must be examined especially carefully. Ultrasonography should be employed in cases in which complete visualization of the retinal periphery is precluded by media opacity. If removal of the hemorrhage is required for adequate fundus visualization to facilitate retinal treatment, then vitrectomy should be performed either prior to cataract surgery or, in cases of dense cataract, concomitant with or immediately following cataract surgery.

A special clinical scenario seen with growing frequency involves the patient born prematurely or who had retinopathy of prematurity (ROP). The syndrome of adult ROP includes early-onset cataracts and associated rhegmatogenous retinal pathology. Among these patients, the reported risk of RRD after cataract surgery approaches 25%. You should ask all patients if they were born early (< 32 weeks of gestational age) or if they were told that they were born with a low birth weight. Many patients with a history of premature birth or ROP have a myopic refraction, but may not necessarily have posterior cicatricial changes.

Macular edema following cataract surgery or YAG laser capsulotomy typically arises from leakage of fluid from hyperpermeable parafoveal capillaries.[3] This hyperpermeability can be exacerbated by 2 mechanisms: (1) vitreomacular traction and (2) inflammation. Thus, treatment directed at retinal conditions that are associated with traction or inflammation should be helpful in reducing the chance of postoperative macular edema.

Retinal or systemic conditions that signal a high risk for postoperative macular edema include:

- Disorders of the vitreomacular interface (vitreomacular adhesion, posterior hyaloidal contraction, epiretinal membrane). Treatment with topical non-steroidal anti-inflammatory drugs (NSAIDs) beginning 3 to 7 days prior to cataract extraction may reduce the incidence of pseudophakic macular edema and optimize postoperative vision recovery.[4,5] In certain cases of coexisting cataract and vitreomacular interface disease, it is unclear how much of the vision impairment is due to cataract and how much is due to macular disease. In such cases, it is advisable to remove the cataract first, allow complete recovery, and then reassess the extent of macula-related vision impairment.

- The incidence of macular edema following even uneventful cataract surgery is higher in a diabetic eye, even in the absence of diabetic retinopathy, than in nondiabetic eyes.[6] Collective laboratory and clinical evidence suggests a pathoetiologic role for inflammation mediated by prostaglandins and inflammatory cytokines and for vascular permeability driven by vascular endothelial growth factor (VEGF). In 2 prospective, randomized, vehicle-controlled, comparative studies of patients with diabetic retinopathy, treatment with the topical NSAID nepafenac 0.1% (3 times daily, starting 1 day before cataract surgery) was associated with less postoperative macular edema and better visual acuity at 3 months (Table 42-1).[7]

The risk and severity of postoperative macular edema and the risk of exacerbating diabetic retinopathy are correlated with the severity of macular edema and diabetic retinopathy at the time of cataract surgery. While the conventional teaching has been to control diabetic retinopathy and eradicate macular edema (traditionally using laser photocoagulation) completely for several months prior to cataract surgery, this may not always be achievable, and the time required to do so may delay the time to vision improvement. Intravitreal administration of corticosteroid (typically in the form of triamcinolone or a Ozurdex implant [dexamethasone]) and/or anti-VEGF medications (eg, bevacizumab, ranibizumab, aflibercept) significantly reduce

Table 42-1

Recommendations for Perioperative Pharmacologic Treatment in Patients With Retinal Vascular Disease Undergoing Cataract Surgery

Topical NSAID	• All diabetic eyes
Intravitreal anti-VEGF and corticosteroid	• Diabetic macular edema • History of diabetic retinopathy in which cataract precludes macular examination
Intravitreal anti-VEGF	• Severe nonproliferative diabetic retinopathy • Proliferative diabetic retinopathy PDR • History of PDR • Significant peripheral capillary nonperfusion • Retinal vein occlusion with macular edema • Retinal vein occlusion with recent treatment for macular edema

postoperative macular edema in diabetic eyes (see Table 42-1).[8] A special situation involves the patient with longstanding (typically several decades) or chronically poorly controlled diabetes in whom minimal or no retinopathy is seen. In such cases of silent retinopathy or featureless retina, chronic retinal ischemia has damaged the native retinal vasculature so severely that the typical compensatory microaneurymal and neovascular changes cannot arise. Fluorescein angiography reveals massive peripheral capillary nonperfusion. When unrecognized and untreated, these eyes can progress rapidly to neovascular glaucoma within a short time following cataract surgery. Prophylactic treatment with anti-VEGF medication and/or panretinal laser photocoagulation is recommended in such cases.

- As in diabetic retinopathy, retinal ischemia arising from venous occlusion can lead to vision-threatening macular edema or vitreous hemorrhage due to posterior segment neovascularization. These complications are mediated primarily by increased VEGF levels driven by retinal ischemia. Perioperative treatment with anti-VEGF medications is recommended in eyes with macular edema or in eyes recently treated for macular edema (see Table 42-1). In eyes with vitreous hemorrhage due to neovascularization, preoperative peripheral scatter retinal laser photocoagulation to the affected area is recommended.

Oh! And What About Timing of the Anti-VEGF Injection?

The goal of perioperative anti-VEGF treatment is to suppress excessive levels of VEGF at the time of, and immediately following, cataract surgery. One wants the highest concentration of anti-VEGF medication at the time of surgery. Pharmacokinetic and clinical data suggest that these peak levels occur, and therapeutic effect begins, at 3 to 7 days following intravitreal injection.

By performing the anti-VEGF injection about 1 week prior to cataract surgery, the complications of intravitreal injection that may interfere with, or further complicate cataract surgery, most notably infectious endophthalmitis or severe noninfectious inflammation, will have already occurred, if they were going to happen. Typically, symptoms of inflammation develop within several days following intravitreal injection. Though these complications are uncommon, it may be preferable to pass safely through this risk period before performing cataract surgery.

Taken together, therefore, the ideal timing of anti-VEGF injection is about 1 week prior to cataract surgery.

In some cases, however, for practical reasons relating to scheduling efficiency, access challenges, or patient compliance, anti-VEGF injection can be performed at the immediate conclusion of cataract extraction under sterile operative conditions.

References

1. Lois N, Wong D. Pseudophakic retinal detachment. *Surv Ophthalmol.* 2003;48(5):467-487.
2. Fincham GS, Pasea L, Carroll C, et al. Prevention of retinal detachment in Stickler syndrome: the Cambridge prophylactic cryotherapy protocol. *Ophthalmology.* 2014;121(8):1588-1597.
3. Chu CJ, Johnston RL, Buscombe C, et al. Risk factors and incidence of macular edema after cataract surgery: a database study of 81984 eyes. *Ophthalmology.* 2016;123(2):316-323.
4. Lim BX, Lim CH, Lim DK, et al. Prophylactic non-steroidal anti-inflammatory drugs for the prevention of macular oedema after cataract surgery. *Cochrane Database Syst Rev.* 2016;11:CD006683.
5. McCafferty S, Harris A, Kew C, et al. Pseudophakic cystoid macular edema prevention and risk factors; prospective study with adjunctive once daily topical nepafenac 0.3% versus placebo. *BMC Ophthalmol.* 2017;17(1):16.
6. Wielders LH, Lambermont VA, Schouten JS, et al Prevention of cystoid macular edema after cataract surgery in nondiabetic and diabetic patients: a systematic review and meta-analysis. *Am J Ophthalmol.* 2015;160(5):968-981.
7. Singh RP, Staurenghi G, Pollack A, et al. Efficacy of nepafenac ophthalmic suspension 0.1% in improving clinical outcomes following cataract surgery in patients with diabetes: an analysis of two randomized studies. *Clin Ophthalmol.* 2017;11:1021-1029.
8. Boscia F, Giancipoli E, D'Amico Ricci G, Pinna A. Management of macular oedema in diabetic patients undergoing cataract surgery. *Curr Opin Ophthalmol.* 2017;28(1):23-28.

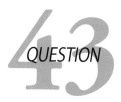

QUESTION

DO CHRONIC RHEGMATOGENOUS RETINAL DETACHMENTS NEED SURGICAL REPAIR?

Charles C. Wykoff, MD, PhD
Harry W. Flynn, Jr., MD
Nidhi Relhan Batra, MD

Rhegmatogenous retinal detachment (RRD) is a frequent clinical challenge affecting approximately 1/200 people over the course of a lifetime.[1] An RRD is one of the most common indications for vitreoretinal surgery and such surgical repair is one of the most cost-effective practices in the treatment of vitreoretinal disorders.[2,3] Despite this, some asymptomatic chronic RRDs may be observed and may not progress.[4,5]

Two key factors should be considered when determining if serial observation may be a reasonable approach to the management of a chronic RRD.

First, while there are many points to consider in the patient history, perhaps the most important is the presence or absence of symptoms. In many fields of medicine, patients with the same clinical problem, one symptomatic and the other asymptomatic, may be treated quite differently; for example, in the settings of cholelithiasis where the presence of symptoms may indicate intervention that otherwise may have been deferred. While self-evident, it is worth recognizing that in the absence of current or past symptoms, it is not possible to make a patient symptomatically better. In the setting of an individual without the expected capacity to recognize or report symptoms, however, this factor is less important and possibly irrelevant. Asymptomatic RRD suggests an absence of tractional forces on the retinal break or lack of an acute posterior vitreous detachment (PVD). Published reports indicate that an asymptomatic RRD can sometimes progress slowly, but good anatomic and visual outcomes can still be achieved with surgical intervention if ultimately necessary (Table 43-1).[6-10] For example, Kothari and colleagues [10] reported 3 patients with chronic RRDs associated with subretinal bands successfully repaired with good visual outcomes.

Fekrat S, ed. *Curbside Consultation in Retina: 49 Clinical Questions, Second Edition.* (pp 219-223).
© 2019 SLACK Incorporated

Table 43-1

Retrospective Series Reporting Anatomic and Visual Outcomes Following Surgical Management of Asymptomatic RRDs After the Retinal Detachment Progressed or the Patient Became Symptomatic

	n/N (eyes)	Rx	Anatomical Success (%)	Key Findings
Tillery et al (1976)[6]	60/60	SB: All	98% eyes	• 15% had worse VA postoperatively
Benson et al (1977)[7]	66/66	SB: All	98.5% eyes	• 51/66 eyes had progression despite demarcation lines
Jarret et al (1988)[8]	8/16	SB: 8	100% eyes	• 8/16 eyes did not progress
Brod et al (1995)[9]	2/31	SB: 2	100% eyes	• Postoperative VA: 20/20 both cases • 52% did not have PVD
Kothari et al (2016)[10]	3/3	SB: All	100% eyes	• Postoperative VA: 20/25, 20/50 and 20/20

SB = scleral buckle; VA = visual acuity; n = number of eyes where asymptomatic rhegmatogenous retinal detachment progressed; N = total number of eyes

Second, ophthalmoscopic characteristics are important to consider when determining appropriate management. For example, a bullous, fovea-threatening, superior RRD in the setting of an acute PVD is a clear indication for urgent surgical repair. In contrast, an asymptomatic, shallow, peripheral RRD secondary to an atrophic hole within an area of lattice degeneration, lack of PVD, thinned detached retina with intraretinal cysts and demarcation lines, in a non-myopic patient may not require any surgical intervention (Figures 43-1 through 43-3). Other anatomic factors to consider include macula status, presence of a retinal dialysis, and lens status. Preexisting poor function of the macula in an eye with a chronic macula-involving RRD may be observed in select circumstances. An asymptomatic chronic RRD in an eye with an inferior retinal dialysis may not progress for many years since subretinal fluid may accumulate very slowly.[4] Nonprogression of chronic asymptomatic RRD has been well-documented in both phakic and aphakic eyes.[11,12]

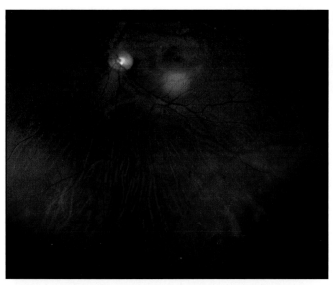

Figure 43-1. Asymptomatic, shallow, peripheral, inferior, RRD secondary to atrophic retinal holes within an area of lattice degeneration with associated thinning of the detached retina in the setting of an attached vitreous.

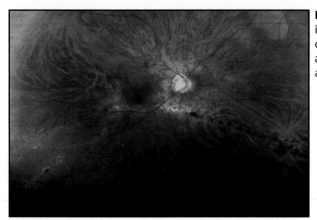

Figure 43-2. Asymptomatic, shallow, inferior RRD with a prominent pigmentary demarcation line at the superior border and subretinal bands in the setting of an attached vitreous.

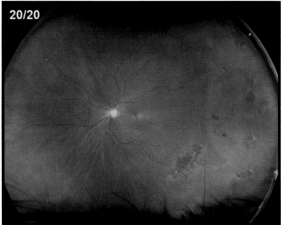

Figure 43-3. Fundus photograph of the left eye of a 59-year-old female showing chronic, temporal retinal detachment associated with atrophic retinal holes and pigmentary changes. The patient has remained asymptomatic, with stable best-corrected visual acuity (20/20) and stable borders of the retinal detachment over 5 years of follow-up.

In general, a symptomatic RRD is cause for intervention, either aimed at retinal reattachment or aimed at cessation of progression. Excellent outcomes may be obtained with retinal reattachment surgery using 3 distinct approaches: scleral buckling, pars plana vitrectomy, and/or pneumatic retinopexy. In some clinical situations, however, especially RRD that are small, shallow, and peripheral, demarcation laser photocoagulation intended not to reattach the retina but rather to stop expansion of the RRD may be a reasonable alternative.[13]

In comparison, some asymptomatic RRDs may be serially observed without intervention. Asymptomatic RRDs account for less than 5% of all RRD.[4] Subclinical RRDs are often asymptomatic. In 1973, Davis defined subclinical RRD as an RRD extending at least 1 disc diameter from a retinal break but no more than 2 disc diameters posterior to the equator.[14] Such asymptomatic RRDs are commonly caused by atrophic holes in lattice degeneration and are often located in inferior quadrants.[15]

Demarcation lines are an important clinical finding that we look for to signify chronicity. In a prospective study of 18 consecutive asymptomatic RRDs, 100% had at least a partial demarcation line, none became symptomatic over an average of 46 months of follow-up, and only 1 showed progression of its border.[16] Many subclinical RRDs have demonstrated clinical stability for many months to years without progression and without the development of symptoms.[4] It is important to note that demarcation lines indicate chronicity of the RRD but do not necessarily restrict the spread of subretinal fluid.[7,9]

Regardless of what treatment—if any—is pursued, we find patient education to be a critical component of management. While many subclinical, asymptomatic RRDs will remain stable for an extended period, some will progress. Patients need to be aware of this possibility, understand the risks and benefits of both observation and intervention, and agree to the management plan. While well-meaning, surgical intervention aimed at retinal reattachment can have untoward effects including cataract acceleration, glaucoma, infection, bleeding, cystoid macular edema, diplopia, refractive shift, and the development of proliferative vitreoretinopathy, which can ultimately lead to a poorer visual outcome. If serial observation is agreed upon, we review steps for monocular self-monitoring of the visual field with the patient and develop a management plan if progression is noted.

There are certain clinical scenarios that increase our likelihood of intervening in an eye with an asymptomatic, subclinical RRD. First, in those patients with an asymptomatic RRD in one eye and a history of a repaired RRD in the fellow eye, surgical repair of the asymptomatic RRD should be considered. Second, the patient's activities and profession should be considered. Direct trauma to the head and periocular tissues from sports, such as boxing, martial arts, and any other activity that may lead to head trauma is a recognized risk factor for RRD development and possible progression. Surgical intervention may be indicated in such individuals with an asymptomatic RRD. Third, timely access to health care should be considered. Reliable, consistent, serial examinations are warranted in the setting of an asymptomatic RRD that is being observed, because if substantial progression of the border is noted, even in the continued absence of symptoms, intervention may be indicated. Finally, specific ocular characteristics may increase the likelihood of intervention including extensive location, high myopia, superior and bullous characteristics, and absence of a demarcation line.

Additional common clinical scenarios involving patients with asymptomatic RRD include patients undergoing planned ocular interventions including cataract surgery, yttrium-aluminum-garnet laser capsulotomy, and refractive surgery. These and other ocular procedures may carry an increased risk of RRD. Furthermore, eyes undergoing such interventions may be at elevated risk of an RRD compared to the general population. For example, increased myopia has been correlated with an increased risk of RRD. Therefore, specific patient education related to any additional risk factors must be considered and management decisions should be individualized.

Summary

The presentation of an asymptomatic RRD requires an individualized approach. In the setting of an asymptomatic, small, peripheral RRD with a demarcation line in a reliable patient without other external risk factors, serial clinical observations may be considered as a reasonable management option.

References

1. Sodhi A, Leung LS, Do DV, et al. Recent trends in the management of rhegmatogenous retinal detachment. *Surv Ophthalmol*. 2008;53(1):50-67.
2. Chang JS, Smiddy WE. Cost-effectiveness of retinal detachment repair. *Ophthalmology*. 2014;121(4):946-951.
3. Wykoff CC, Flynn HW Jr, Scott IU. What is the optimal timing for rhegmatogenous retinal detachment repair? *JAMA Ophthalmol*. 2013;131(11):1399-1400.
4. Brod RD, Flynn HW, Jr. Asymptomatic rhegmatogenous retinal detachment. *Curr Opin Ophthalmol*. 1996;7(3):1-6.
5. Byer NE. Spontaneous regression and disappearance of subclinical rhegmatogenous retinal detachment. *Am J Ophthalmol*. 2001;131(2):269-270.
6. Tillery WV, Lucier AC. Round atrophic holes in lattice degeneration--an important cause of phakic retinal detachment. *Trans Sect Ophthalmol Am Acad Ophthalmol Otolaryngol*. 1976;81(3 Pt 1):509-518.
7. Benson WE, Nantawan P, Morse PH. Characteristics and prognosis of retinal detachments with demarcation lines. *Am J Ophthalmol*. 1977;84(5):641-644.
8. Jarrett WH II. Retinal detachment: is reparative surgery always mandatory? *Trans Am Ophthalmol Soc*. 1988;86:307-320.
9. Brod RD, Flynn HW Jr, Lightman DA. Asymptomatic rhegmatogenous retinal detachments. *Arch Ophthalmol*. 1995;113(8):1030-10322.
10. Kothari N, Kuriyan AE, Flynn HW, Jr. Spectral domain optical coherence tomography imaging of subretinal bands associated with chronic retinal detachments. *Clin Ophthalmol*. 2016;10:467-470.
11. Friedman Z, Neumann E. Posterior vitreous detachment after cataract extraction in non-myopic eyes and the resulting retinal lesions. *Br J Ophthalmol*. 1975;59(8):451-454.
12. Byer NE. The natural history of asymptomatic retinal breaks. *Ophthalmology*. 1982;89(9):1033-1039.
13. Vrabec TR, Baumal CR. Demarcation laser photocoagulation of selected macula-sparing rhegmatogenous retinal detachments. *Ophthalmology*. 2000;107(6):1063-1067.
14. Davis MD. The natural history of retinal breaks without detachment. *Trans Am Ophthalmol Soc*. 1973;71:343-372.
15. Byer NE. Long-term natural history of lattice degeneration of the retina. *Ophthalmology*. 1989;96(9):1396-401; discussion 401-402.
16. Cohen SM. Natural history of asymptomatic clinical retinal detachments. *Am J Ophthalmol*. 2005;139(5):777-779.

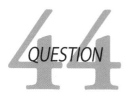

SHOULD I USE JETREA OR A GAS BUBBLE OR JUST DO A VITRECTOMY FOR A VITREOMACULAR TRACTION?

Michael N. Cohen, MD

Caroline R. Baumal, MD

In 2013, the International Vitreomacular Traction Study Group introduced an optical coherence tomography (OCT)-based classification system to characterize the vitreomacular interface (VMI) (Table 44-1).[1] The term vitreomacular adhesion (VMA) defines non-pathological perifoveal vitreous separation with residual vitreomacular attachment and preserved foveal architecture (Figure 44-1). In contrast, vitreomacular traction (VMT) is a pathological state defined on OCT by persistent vitreous attachment inducing anatomic distortion of the fovea (Figure 44-2). Full-thickness macular hole (FTMH) demonstrates central interruption of all retinal layers on OCT and is classified as primary (due to VMT) or secondary (resulting from another pathologic process) and subclassified by size as small (≤250 μm), medium (>250 and ≤400 μm), or large (>400 μm) and by the presence or absence of concurrent VMT. Use of this classification system across clinical trials has allowed analysis of medical and surgical treatment options for VMT and FTMH.

The initial step when evaluating a patient with VMT is to assess visual acuity and symptoms. Patients who are truly symptomatic by VMT complain of metamorphopsia or central blurred vision, often stating that they have to close the affected eye when reading or driving. If the patient is asymptomatic and/or visual acuity is 20/40 or better, observation may be indicated with periodic re-evaluation for a drop in visual acuity or the onset of symptoms. Individuals with reduced acuity and/or symptomatic metamorphopsia should be presented with the available options, including observation, intravitreal Jetrea (ocriplasmin), intravitreal injection of an expansile gas bubble, or pars plana vitrectomy (PPV). Even for those who are symptomatic, it is reasonable to offer a brief period of observation using OCT to track for potential changes. The natural history of VMT is variable (see Figure 44-2). It can persist with a stable level of retinal disruption or it may progress

Fekrat S, ed. *Curbside Consultation in Retina: 49 Clinical Questions, Second Edition.* (pp 225-229).
© 2019 SLACK Incorporated

Table 44-1

Optical Coherence Tomography of the Vitreomacular Interface

Vitreomacular Interface Finding	Optical Coherence Tomography Finding
VMA	Evidence of perifoveal vitreous detachment from the retinal surface with residual macular attachment and no change in foveal contour or retinal architecture
VMT	Evidence of perifoveal vitreous detachment from the retinal surface with residual macular attachment with associated distortion of foveal surface or retinal architecture
FTMH	Full-thickness foveal interruption from the ILM to RPE
LMH	Irregular foveal contour with inner retinal defect, or splitting, but intact outer retina/ellipsoid zone
Macular Pseudohole	Heaped foveal edges with concomitant ERM with no loss of retinal tissue

ILM = internal limiting membrane; RPE = retinal pigment epithelium; ERM = epiretinal membrane; LMH = lamellar macular hole

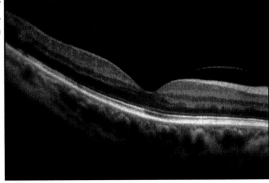

Figure 44-1. Spectral domain optical coherence tomography (SD-OCT) demonstrating VMA, which can be classified as focal or broad. This is a non-pathological finding.

with increased retinal distortion or develop into a FTMH. Spontaneous release of VMT may also occur, leading to either complete resolution of VMT or development of a FTMH. Rates of spontaneous resolution of VMT are not universally agreed upon, but reported release rates have ranged from 6% to 10% over a 1-month period to 17% to 32% over 18 to 24 months.[2] Close follow-up over weeks to months can allow a patient to consider all options and make an informed decision, while at the same time observing for potential spontaneous resolution of traction.

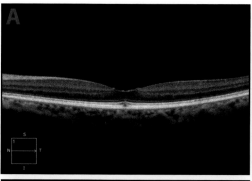

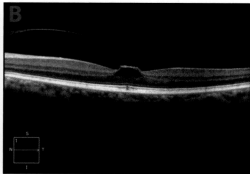

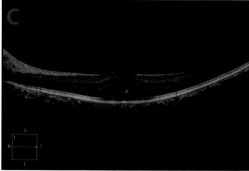

Figure 44-2. Natural history: Progression of VMT to FTMH. (A) Focal VMT demonstrated on SD-OCT with mild disruption of the inner retinal contour. Visual acuity was 20/25. (B) Progression VMT with inner retinal pseudocysts. Visual acuity declined to 20/30. (C) Progression of VMT into a small FTMH. Visual acuity further declined to 20/70.

For many years, surgical intervention with PPV had been the cornerstone of VMT treatment. In late 2012, the US Food and Drug Administration–approved the intravitreal injection of ocriplasmin for the treatment of VMT based on results from 2 Phase III clinical trials. This recombinant protease achieves vitreomacular release through its proteolytic activity against laminin and fibronectin—2 key components of the vitreoretinal interface. Two Phase III trials, the MIVI-TRUST (Microplasmin for Intravitreal Injection-Traction Release Without Surgical Treatment) and OASIS (Ocriplasmin for Treatment for Symptomatic Vitreomacular Adhesion Including Macular Hole) demonstrated efficacy of this non-surgical option, with an increased rate of vitreomacular release at day 28 (26.5% vs 10.1% in MIVI-TRUST and 41.7% vs. 6.2% in OASIS) compared to eyes receiving placebo/sham injection. Only MIVI-TRUST showed a statistically significant improvement in visual acuity at 6 months in eyes treated with ocriplasmin compared to eyes that received sham/placebo. Eyes with good visual acuity (20/25 or better in MIVI-TRUST; 20/30 or better in OASIS) and eyes with large FTMH (> 400 µm) were excluded from both studies. There are some concerning serious, albeit rarely reported, adverse events associated with use of ocriplasmin, including decreased visual acuity, OCT ellipsoid zone disruption, development of subfoveal fluid, electroretinogram changes, retinal break and detachment, lens subluxation or instability, dyschromatopsia, and abnormal pupillary reflex. In most cases, these adverse events have been temporary and a good visual outcome was ultimately obtained, but there have been select reports of permanent scotoma and visual loss.

Despite the intrigue of a pharmacologic option to address VMT, the only modest success rates, high cost, and risk of permanent adverse events have left many in the retina community hesitant to use ocriplasmin. Pneumatic vitreolysis, in which an expansile gas bubble (C_3F_8 or SF_6) is injected into the vitreous cavity to induce a complete posterior vitreous detachment, is much less invasive than PPV. It is hypothesized that the buoyant force induced by the gas bubble causes a mechanical separation of the vitreoretinal interface. The procedure was initially described in the early 1990s as an alternative to vitrectomy to close macular holes. It most commonly involves the injection of 0.30 mL of gas 3.5 to 4 mm posterior to the limbus, preceded by an anterior chamber paracentesis. Four

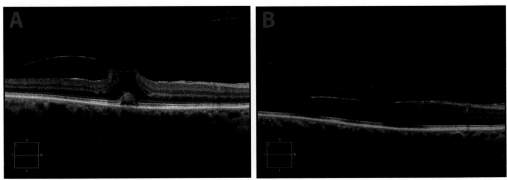

Figure 44-3. (A) VMT on SD-OCT. Visual acuity was 20/70 with metamorphopsia. (B) Resolution of VMT after PPV. Visual acuity improved to 20/30 4 weeks postoperatively. A subtle ERM is noted on the inner retina surface.

retrospective, non-randomized, small case series have reported impressive rates of VMT release at 1-month post-injection.[3] Complications reported were rare and included development of a retinal break, progression to a macular hole, transient ellipsoid zone changes on OCT, and an episode of pupillary block. While there is early evidence to suggest that pneumatic vitreolysis may be an effective option to treat VMT, it is premature to interpret the rates of release (or complications) on such a small total sample size of only 74 total patients without a fully randomized, controlled, prospective trial.

The most effective and reliable method to relieve VMT remains PPV (Figure 44-3). The rate of VMT release after PPV is reported at over 90%, but found to be even higher in clinical practice.[4] More recent surgical reports suggest that 95% of patients with VMT have improved visual acuity after PPV, with 45% achieving an improvement of greater than 2 lines.[5] During vitrectomy, the ability to remove the cortical vitreous, remove any potential ERM, and peel the internal limiting membrane is the most complete way to relieve both anterior-posterior and tangential traction on the macula. The current era of small gauge vitrectomy surgery has improved both safety and outcomes, and such a surgical approach has the longest track record for treating VMT. Progression of cataract may occur after PPV, which can affect postoperative visual acuity results in any case series evaluating PPV for VMT. It is important to inform phakic patients that their cataract may progress after PPV in the surgical eye eventually necessitating surgical removal. With PPV, the risk of endophthalmitis is quite low, at around 0.01%. It appears that the risk of a retinal break after any of the aforementioned treatment options is around 1% and is likely related to the pathophysiology of VMT with its associated abnormally tight vitreoretinal adherence.

Table 44-2
Current Treatment Options for Vitreomacular Traction
• Observation • Intravitreal injection of ocriplasmin • Intravitreal injection of expansile gas • PPV

For symptomatic patients with VMT, the most successful treatment both anatomically and visually is currently vitrectomy. Ocriplasmin and pneumatic vitreolysis remain options; however, one must be prepared for vitrectomy if these less invasive options are not successful. As spontaneous resolution is part of the natural history of VMT, it is important to include a control group when evaluating pharmacologic treatment for VMT (Table 44-2). Further clinical studies are needed to characterize eyes that will respond to pneumatic vitreolysis. To maximize gains in visual acuity, it is likely best not to wait to more than several months before intervention.

References

1. Duker JS, Kaiser PK, Binder S, et al. The International Vitreomacular Traction Study Group classification of vitreomacular adhesion, traction, and macular hole. *Ophthalmology.* 2013;120(12):2611–2619.
2. Stalmans P, Benz MS, Gandorfer A,et al; MIVI-TRUST Study Group. Enzymatic vitreolysis with ocriplasmin for vitreomacular traction and macular holes. *N Engl J Med.* 2012;367(7):606-615.
3. Steinle NC, Dhoot DS, Quezada Ruiz C, et al. Treatment of vitreomacular traction with intravitreal perfluoropropane (C3F8) injection. *Retina.* 2017;37(4):643-650.
4. Gonzalez MA, Flynn HW Jr, Bokman CM, Feuer W, Smiddy WE. Outcomes of pars plana vitrectomy for patients with vitreomacular traction. *Ophthalmic Surg Lasers Imaging Retina.* 2015;46(7):708-714
5. Witkin AJ, Patron ME, Castro LC, et al. Anatomic and visual outcomes of vitrectomy for vitreomacular traction syndrome. *Ophthalmic Surg Lasers Imaging.* 2010;41(4):425-431.

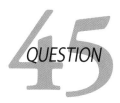

WHEN SHOULD A PATIENT WITH DIABETIC RETINOPATHY BE CONSIDERED FOR A VITRECTOMY?

Ronald C. Gentile MD, FACS, FASRS

Alexander Barash, MD

Diabetic retinopathy is the leading cause of blindness in working-aged persons in the United States.[1] Diabetic vitrectomy is reserved for eyes with complications of diabetic retinopathy not amenable to intravitreal injection or laser. Even among compliant patients with frequent ophthalmic exams and timely scatter panretinal laser photocoagulation, vitrectomy still becomes necessary in at least 5% of patients.[2] The surgical goal of a diabetic vitrectomy is to clear the vitreous of opacities, release and remove tractional elements from the retinal surface, promote attachment or reattach any detached retina, and complete panretinal photocoagulation with or without the addition of intravitreal pharmacological agents.

The 2 predominant classic indications for diabetic vitrectomy, nonclearing vitreous hemorrhage and tractional retinal detachment involving the macula, have remained the same since the results of the Diabetic Retinopathy Vitrectomy Study were published in the 1980s.

We have divided indications for diabetic vitrectomy into 5 broad categories (Table 45-1). These categories include (A) retinal detachment, (B) hemorrhage, (C) severe retinal neovascularization, (D) macular pathology, and (E) postvitrectomy. As it is not uncommon for eyes to have more than one indication for diabetic vitrectomy, a sixth category was added to include F. Combinations of A to E. Most indications are for complications of proliferative diabetic retinopathy (PDR) with a small percentage due to complications of nonproliferative diabetic retinopathy.

Fekrat S, ed. *Curbside Consultation in Retina: 49 Clinical Questions, Second Edition.* (pp 231-237).
© 2019 SLACK Incorporated

Table 45-1
Indications for Diabetic Vitrectomy

A. Retinal detachment
- Tractional retinal detachment involving or threatening the macula
- Combined tractional-rhegmatogenous retinal detachment (RRD)
- RRD

B. Hemorrhage
- Nonclearing vitreous hemorrhage
- Subhyaloid premacular loculated hemorrhage
- Vitreous hemorrhage with anterior segment neovascularization
- Bilateral vitreous hemorrhage
- Subretinal hemorrhage (rare)
- Other vitreous opacities (ie, asteroid hyalosis, amyloidosis, inflammatory cells)

C. Very severe retinal neovascularization and fibrovascular proliferation

D. Macular pathology
- Taut hyaloid
- Premacular fibrosis with or without neovascularization
- Vitreomacular traction syndrome
- Macular hole
- Persistent macular edema

E. Postvitrectomy
- All of the above that apply
- Anterior hyaloidal fibrovascular proliferation
- Fibrinoid syndrome
- Reproliferation of preretinal membranes
- Taut internal limiting membrane (ILM)
- Ghost cell glaucoma

F. Combinations of A through E

A. Retinal Detachment

Tractional retinal detachment (Figure 45-1) involving or threatening the macula is one of the classic indications for diabetic vitrectomy. This usually occurs when retinal neovascularization develops along the vascular arcades with multiple epicenters, becomes fibrotic, and contracts causing the underlying retina to elevate and detach. This can occur with or without a partial posterior vitreous detachment (PVD). Tractional retinal detachment not involving the macula is not an indication for surgery because it can remain stable. This is especially true when the retinal neovascular component is inactive and fibrotic, most often seen after full prior-panretinal laser photocoagulation has been performed. It is important to note that intravitreal injections of anti-vascular endothelial growth factor (anti-VEGF) medications are to be used with caution in eyes with severe PDR especially if there is a tractional detachment near the macula, as they may cause progression of the tractional detachment. Tractional retinal detachments precipitated by an

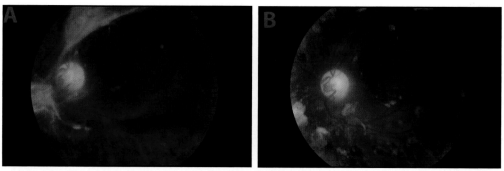

Figure 45-1. (A) Tractional diabetic retinal detachment involving the macula. (B) Two months postdiabetic vitrectomy with removal of the fibrotic neovascularization and release of the traction. The retina subsequently reattached with residual macular transposition.

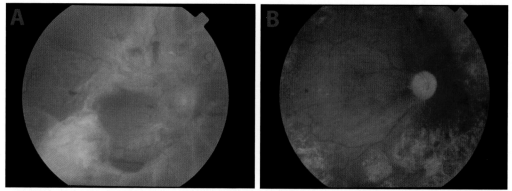

Figure 45-2. (A) Combined diabetic tractional-RRD. Note the outer retinal hydration line over a partially convex surface superiorly. (B) Three months postdiabetic vitrectomy after removal of the fibrotic neovascularization, release of all traction, drainage of fluid from the retinal break, endolaser, and reattachment of the retina using gas tamponade.

intravitreal injection of anti-VEGF generally occur 2 weeks after the injection, but can range from 3 to 21 days.[3] When using preoperative intravitreal anti-VEGF agents before a diabetic vitrectomy with active neovascularization, some authors recommend it be given no more than 5 days preoperatively to avoid progression of the detachment.[4]

Combined tractional-RRDs (Figure 45-2) are usually a result of a partial vitreous detachment in the setting of cicatricial PDR. These detachments can progress very quickly and require extensive hyaloid and membrane removal on a mobile retina to repair. Breaks in tractional-RRDs are usually small and located adjacent to tractionally elevated epicenters posterior to the equator and sometimes at vulnerable areas of old chorioretinal scars. They can also originate from a macular hole. Many breaks are only identified intraoperatively because fibrosis and hemorrhage may prevent preoperative visualization. Unlike purely tractional retinal detachments, tractional-RRDs are more mobile, have outer retinal hydration lines, and a partial convex surface.

RRDs can occur in the setting of diabetic retinopathy, although they are much less common than the aforementioned types. Their management is similar in eyes without retinopathy with particular attention to postoperative worsening of retinopathy and macular edema.

Table 45-2
Vitreous Hemorrhage: Factors That Support Diabetic Vitrectomy

Vitrectomy	No	Yes
Vitreous hemorrhage density	Not severe PRP possible	Severe PRP not possible
B-scan ultrasound	PVD	No PVD Tractional macular elevation
Anterior segment neovascularization	Absent	Present**
Fellow eye	Stable Good vision	Active PDR Poor vision
Diabetes type	Type II	Type I
Prior PRP/Anti-VEGF*	Yes	No
Severe retinal neovascularization	No Inactive	Yes Active

*Multiple and continuous without causing progressive tractional detachment
**Especially if anti-VEGF cannot be given or is contraindicated

B. Hemorrhage

Vitreous hemorrhage is the other classic indication for diabetic vitrectomy, especially when it is visually significant and nonclearing. The hemorrhage is considered visually significant if it is responsible for a vision of less than 20/400 and the opacity prevents laser photocoagulation. To determine if the hemorrhage is nonclearing, the patient would have to give a history of no improvement or be examined without improvement for at least 3 to 4 weeks. When examining a patient with a vitreous hemorrhage, it is important to determine the density of the hemorrhage, the status of the underlying retina by B-scan echography, the presence or absence of anterior segment neovascularization, the status of the fellow eye, the extent of prior panretinal photocoagulation (PRP), and the type of diabetes. Ultrasonography should rule out an RRD or tractional retinal detachment involving the macula that would supersede the vitreous hemorrhage as an indication for prompt diabetic vitrectomy. Reasons for an earlier vitrectomy include vitreous hemorrhage in the fellow eye, Type 1 diabetes without prior PRP and with very active PDR, and anterior segment neovascularization (Table 45-2). Preoperative intravitreal anti-VEGF agents may play a role in the management of such patients, especially in the latter 2 conditions, just as long as the risk of causing progression of a tractional detachment is assessed as mentioned previously.

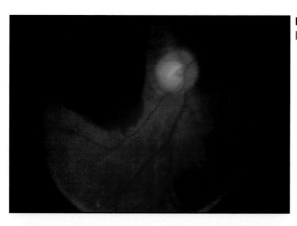

Figure 45-3. Subhyaloid, premacular, loculated hemorrhage.

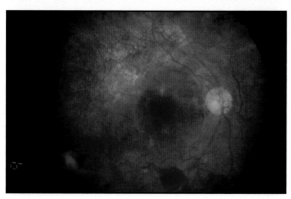

Figure 45-4. Severe retinal neovascularization and fibrovascular proliferation despite PRP.

Subhyaloid premacular, loculated hemorrhage (Figure 45-3), especially when thick and not associated with any progressive detachment of the hyaloid, is an indication for vitrectomy. Dense premacular hemorrhage can lead to progressive fibrosis and, even if it clears, can result in a premacular fibrotic membrane. Subretinal hemorrhage is rare and generally associated with a very adherent and attached hyaloid or retinal break. This is most often only diagnosed intraoperatively.

Other vitreous opacities, when severe enough to prevent diagnosis and treatment of diabetic retinopathy, are a potential indication for vitrectomy. These include the rare case of dense asteroid hyalosis, amyloidosis, or inflammatory cells that can impair fundus visibility for imaging, PRP, and/or other diagnostic and treatment modalities.

C. Very Severe Retinal Neovascularization and Fibrovascular Proliferation

Very severe retinal neovascularization (Figure 45-4) in the presence of an attached hyaloid can extend from the optic nerve to the arcades. The natural history of this process is fibrosis and traction as the neovascularization cicatrizes and results in a broad-based tractional retinal detachment with a tabletop configuration. The tractional detachments can sometimes encircle the macula before the center detaches. These eyes can progress with anti-VEGF treatment, or, despite laser photocoagulation in some cases, the neovascularization can grow over the macula. The prognosis for vision is inversely proportional to the extent of active retinal neovascularization. Vitrectomy in these cases can be difficult and when successful can prevent inevitable blindness.

Figure 45-5. Vitreomacular traction syndrome complicating diabetic retinopathy imaged by optical coherence tomography.

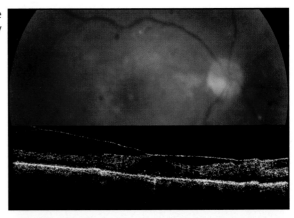

Figure 45-6. Fibrinoid syndrome complicating diabetic vitrectomy. Note the fibrin strands behind an intact peripheral capsule.

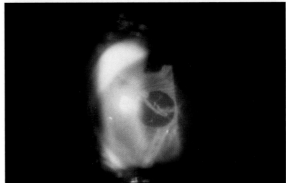

D. Macular Pathology

In a small subset of eyes, a taut hyaloid results in persistent macular edema due to tangential vitreous traction. The macular edema is usually diffuse and removing the hyaloid is very effective in decreasing the edema. Premacular fibrosis with or without neovascularization can occur and in some cases, consists of a fibrotic and contracted hyaloid membrane in front of the macula causing obscuration of the fovea. Vitreomacular traction syndrome (Figure 45-5) can result when the hyaloid remains attached to the fovea or perifoveal region and results in edema and loss of vision. Optical coherence tomography has been very helpful in identifying this condition. Macular holes can occur in the setting of PDR and when associated with extensive fibrovascular proliferation can result in a posterior retinal detachment. Persistent macular edema can be an indication for vitrectomy when all other treatment modalities fail. In these cases, it is felt to be a treatment of last resort by most surgeons, especially with the advent of multiple intravitreal agents.

E. Postvitrectomy

Indications for vitrectomy after an initial diabetic vitrectomy include all of the previously mentioned indications. The most severe indications unique to the postdiabetic vitrectomy eye include anterior hyaloidal fibrovascular proliferation and fibrinoid syndrome (Figure 45-6). Even though less commonly seen today with advances in surgical techniques and the use of adjuvants, these complications typically occur in the most severely affected eyes and, without repeat surgery, these eyes will usually lose light perception and progress to phthisis bulbi. Anterior hyaloidal fibrovascular proliferation presents most commonly with early postoperative vitreous and/or retrolental hemorrhage with extraretinal neovascularization extending from the anterior retina to the anterior hyaloid face and behind the lens.

Fibrinoid syndrome is the most severe form of postvitrectomy fibrin formation with fibrin stands and sheets across the vitreous cavity. Recombinant tissue plasminogen activator can be used to break down the fibrin in the perioperative period. Use of intraoperative and postoperative triamcinolone and/or anti-VEGF agents may decrease the incidence of this complication.

Preretinal reproliferation of membranes can occur after a diabetic vitrectomy and is managed surgically, if severe. In some cases, these membranes can be very adherent and can act as a scaffold for neovascularization in the absence of an intact posterior hyaloid. Taut ILM can cause pharmacologically unresponsive diffuse macular edema with outer retinal edema following a previous diabetic vitrectomy. Tangential tractional forces from contractile cells propagated across the fovea via the ILM appear to be the etiology. Removal of the ILM can restore the normal foveal contour and improve visual acuity in such cases.[5] Ghost cell glaucoma is managed surgically if the intraocular pressure cannot be controlled medically. If most of the vitreous has been previously removed and no other retinal pathology exists, an in-office air-fluid exchange can be performed to remove the bulk of ghost cells and avoid another visit to the operating room. In some cases, intravitreal anti-VEGF may also facilitate clearing.

F. Combinations of A Through E

Many eyes have multiple indications for a diabetic vitrectomy. Some diagnoses have priority over others in the decision regarding the timing of vitrectomy. The higher the risk for progression and irreversible vision loss, the more critical it is that the vitrectomy not be delayed. In general, progressive retinal detachment and medically uncontrollable neovascular glaucoma with media opacities take priority over the other indications.

Summary

Since Machemer's first successful diabetic vitrectomy in the 1970s, we have come a long way in the surgical management of the sequelae associated with PDR. In addition to advances in surgical instrumentation, increased use and study of perioperative, adjuvant, and intravitreal pharmacological therapies are expected as retinal surgeons fine tune their skills in preventing diabetic blindness.

References

1. US Centers for Disease Control and Prevention. *National Diabetes Fact Sheet: General Information and National Estimates on Diabetes in the United States.* Atlanta, GA: Centers for Disease Control and Prevention; 2005.
2. Flynn HW Jr, Chew EY, Simons BD, Barton FB, Remaley NA, Ferris FL III; Early Treatment Diabetic Retinopathy Study Research Group. Pars plana vitrectomy in the Early Treatment Diabetic Retinopathy Study. ETDRS report number 17. *Ophthalmology.* 1992;99:1351-1357.
3. El Rami H, Barham R, Sun JK, Silva PS. Evidence-based treatment of diabetic retinopathy. *Semin Ophthalmol.* 2017;32(1):67-74.
4. Berrocal MH, Acaba LA, Acaba A. Surgery for diabetic eye complications. *Curr Diab Rep.* 2016;16:99.
5. Gentile RC, Milman T, Eliott D, Romero JM, McCormick SA. Taut internal limiting membrane causing diffuse diabetic macular edema after vitrectomy: clinicopathologic correlation. *Ophthalmologica.* 2011;226:64-70.

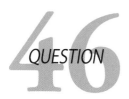

HOW DO I FOLLOW A PATIENT WHO HAS DIABETES AND BECOMES PREGNANT? WHAT TESTS CAN I DO?

Judy E. Kim, MD

Alessa Crossan, MD

Pregnancy complicates the ophthalmic management of patients with preexisting diabetes. Patients who develop gestational diabetes do not develop diabetic retinopathy during pregnancy. Historically, studies have focused on patients with Type 1 diabetes; we presume results can be extrapolated to patients with Type 2 diabetes.

Diabetic retinopathy worsens during pregnancy, although the reasons for this are still debated. Up to 27% of diabetic pregnancies will have diabetic retinopathy at some point.[1] Both clinically significant diabetic macular edema (DME) and proliferative diabetic retinopathy (PDR) may worsen or develop *de novo* during pregnancy.[2,3] Though proliferative disease attracts the most attention, case series have reported severe vision loss from DME.[3] Rates of progression toward PDR have varied widely in the literature. In case series, anywhere from 8% to 70% of patients have shown progression during pregnancy.[1] There is a common and dangerous misconception that retinopathy progression to proliferative disease during pregnancy reverses after delivery. One study found that only 54% of patients improve postpartum,[2] and another detailed a series of patients who demonstrated severe progression following delivery.[4] The risk of progression has been correlated with the duration of diabetes prior to pregnancy, rapid glucose normalization during pregnancy, severity of diabetes at baseline, baseline glycemic control, hypertension, and eclampsia.[2] Therefore, patients with these risk factors should be closely monitored and educated before, during, and even after pregnancy.

Fekrat S, ed. *Curbside Consultation in Retina: 49 Clinical Questions, Second Edition.* (pp 239-242).
© 2019 SLACK Incorporated

How Do I Examine These Patients?

Preconception counseling regarding glycemic control and the potential for progression of diabetic retinopathy is key.[5] Preconception baseline examination is highly recommended to establish the patient's baseline diabetic retinopathy. The actual clinical examination should be equivalent for pregnant and non-pregnant diabetic patients. This should include examination of visual acuity, intraocular pressure, and a thorough anterior segment examination with gonioscopy if necessary to evaluate for neovascularization of the iris and angle. A dilated fundus examination is necessary, since undilated examination may fail to diagnose up to 50% of cases of diabetic retinopathy.[6] Dilating agents, such as cyclopentolate, tropicamide, and phenylephrine, are category C for use in pregnancy, although used frequently with no reported evidence of adverse events for the pregnant patient or the fetus. Nonetheless, it may be prudent to use lower concentrations or to consider punctal occlusion to reduce systemic exposure to these drugs.

Regarding ancillary tests, fundus photography and optical coherence tomography (OCT) clearly pose no adverse risk to the pregnancy. Fundus photography may have varying levels of sensitivity and specificity for detection of retinopathy depending on imaging modality, patient cooperation, and the photographer. There has been an increased use of ultra-widefield fundus photographs in recent years, and it is a good way to noninvasively, quickly, and easily detect, document, and monitor posterior pole disease as well as peripheral lesions. Widefield red free or autofluorescence images may highlight areas of retinal neovascularization. OCT images are the best way to detect even the most subtle intraretinal or subretinal fluid due to DME and help determine areas and the magnitude of retinal thickening. Treatment of DME is often guided by OCT images both in pregnant and non-pregnant diabetic patients, given its noninvasiveness, rapid image capture, quantitative and qualitative information, and registration of images that allow comparison between visits and treatment effects.

While fluorescein angiography (FA) is helpful to evaluate areas of vascular abnormalities, such as microaneurysms, leakage, nonperfusion, and neovascularization, it is usually not performed on pregnant patients due to unknown effects on the fetus. Even in non-pregnant patients, FA is not benign because there is a 1/200,000 chance of a serious adverse event or death.[6] Fluorescein dye has no known risks or teratogenic effects in pregnancy, but neither has it been conclusively determined to be safe. Fortunately, FA is not absolutely necessary to diagnose or treat diabetic retinopathy. It is possible that newer noninvasive imaging modalities, such as OCT angiography, may play a role in assessment and treatment of diabetic patients in the future.

How Often Do I Follow These Patients?

It would be best for any diabetic patients who are contemplating pregnancy to have a baseline ocular examination prior to conception to determine presence of any treatable diabetic retinopathy. This will allow safe use of various agents and treatment modalities without the added concern for the fetus. After the baseline examination prior to conception that incorporates any necessary care, an eye examination during the first trimester is usually recommended.[5] Subsequent follow-up visits depend on the assessed risk of progression based on the severity of retinopathy. Several different follow-up schedules have been suggested in the literature. Second and third trimester examinations are recommended by health organizations in most countries; frequency of exam is dictated by severity and presence of retinopathy.

The most recent publication of the "Preferred Practice Patterns" by the American Academy of Ophthalmology for diabetic retinopathy suggests that pregnant patients found on initial exam to have no retinopathy to mild or moderate nonproliferative diabetic retinopathy (NPDR) have examinations every 3 to 12 months; patients with severe NPDR or worse may need examination every 1 to 3 months.[6] Other sources suggest at least every 3 months[7] or every 4 to 6 weeks.[8] Interestingly, some case series in the literature have followed patients every 2 weeks.[1,4] Follow-up should continue in the postpartum period as well.[1]

Both proliferative disease and any retinopathy with DME require attention during pregnancy. Case series by Rahman and colleagues[1] and Chan and colleagues[4] suggest a cautious follow-up schedule. Patients with more severe disease at baseline were more likely to progress and progressed earlier in their pregnancy. Those with no retinopathy had a 9% rate of progression, while those with early, untreated proliferative disease had a 75% rate of progression. Prior treatment did not completely safeguard against progression; 1 of 4 patients with prior panretinal photocoagulation required further treatment. Rahman and colleagues[1] do concede that their study population probably had a lower rate of treatment compliance and pregestational diabetic care than other groups in the literature. Chan and colleagues[4] specifically looked at patients with progression of retinopathy. The key conclusion one can draw from their paper is to treat pregnant patients with proliferative disease and even those with severe NPDR with laser photocoagulation, as it will likely progress during pregnancy and may not regress after delivery, leading to extremely poor visual outcomes.[4] The concept that those with minimal baseline diabetic retinopathy are unlikely to progress to visually threatening changes and those with moderate to more severe retinopathy are at higher risk of sight threatening progression has been borne out by other cohort studies as well.[9,10] The natural history of DME in pregnancy has not been well studied. The possibility for spontaneous remission after delivery implies less urgency relative to proliferative disease.[11]

How Do I Treat These Patients?

As in all diabetic patients, optimal systemic management of blood pressure, blood sugar, and lipids is essential. Laser photocoagulation is the mainstay of treatment for diabetic retinopathy in pregnant patients due to no known adverse effects on the fetus, with the same protocols and indications as for non-pregnant diabetic patients.[5] While some have used intravitreal injections of steroids for management of severe DME during pregnancy, given theoretical safety, there is very little information in the literature regarding its use during pregnancy. Steroids available for use in the eye for treatment of DME include off-label use of Kenalog (triamcinolone acetate), off-label use of preservative-free Triesence (triamcinolone acetonide), on-label use of Ozurdex implant (dexamethasone), and on-label use of Iluvien implant (fluocinolone). However, these drugs are all category C for use during pregnancy. A recent case series reports use of a dexamethasone implant for management of DME in 5 pregnant patients with improvement in vision and no known complications to the baby.[12] However, the follow-up was limited to the immediate postpartum period.[9] Further reports on the use of these drugs in pregnancy will likely guide subsequent treatment recommendations.

Anti-vascular endothelial growth factor (anti-VEGF) agents such as Avastin (bevacizumab), Lucentis (ranibizumab), and Eylea (aflibercept) are currently the first-line treatment for eyes with DME. They can be also used for the treatment of proliferative disease in diabetic patients. Because all these medications are Category C for use during pregnancy, current literature on the use of anti-VEGF agents in pregnancy is quite limited. Reports exist of miscarriage and preeclampsia after use of bevacizumab; however, the paucity of cases limits our understanding of anti-VEGF's adverse effects.[13] Currently, pregnancy is a contraindication for anti-VEGF agents in our practice due to safety concerns. It may be prudent to consider pregnancy testing in women of child bearing age who are starting anti-VEGF treatment. Review of published cases of anti-VEGF therapy and pregnancy indicates 50% of women discovered that they were pregnant only after anti-VEGF treatment was initiated.[11]

Surgical intervention with pars plana vitrectomy and membrane peeling is an option in select cases for macula—threatening or involving retinal detachment or severe nonclearing vitreous hemorrhage. However, the risk to the mother and fetus must be carefully considered, with the input from other specialists involved in their care. Naturally, surgery would always be viewed as the last option and, if possible, avoided until after delivery. It is hoped that with optimal prenatal care, eye examinations, and timely treatment as outlined in the beginning of this chapter, these eyes would not progress to advanced retinopathy requiring surgery. With a team approach among the various specialists caring for the pregnant diabetic patient, we can improve the visual outcome of the mother while protecting the baby.

References

1. Rahman W, Rahman FZ, Yassin S, Al-Suleiman SA, Rahman J. Progression of retinopathy during pregnancy in type 1 diabetes mellitus. *Clin Experiment Ophthalmol.* 2007;35(3):231-236.
2. Soubrane G, Coscas G. Influence of pregnancy on the evolution of diabetic retinopathy. *Int Ophthalmol Clin.* 1998;38(2):187-194.
3. Sinclair SH, Nesler C, Foxman B, Nichols CW, Gabbe S. Macular edema and pregnancy in insulin-dependent diabetes. *Am J Ophthalmol.* 1984;97(2):154-167.
4. Chan WC, Lim LT, Quinn MJ, Knox FA, McCance D, Best RM. Management and outcome of sight-threatening diabetic retinopathy in pregnancy. *Eye.* 2004;18(8):826-832.
5. Morrison JL, Hodgson LA, Lim LL, Al-Qureshi S. Diabetic retinopathy in pregnancy: a review. *Clin Exp Ophthalmol.* 2016; 44:321-334.
6. American Academy of Ophthalmology Retina Panel. *Preferred Practice Pattern: Diabetic Retinopathy.* San Francisco, CA: American Academy of Ophthalmology; 2016.
7. American Academy of Ophthalmology. *Basic and Clinical Science Course: Retina and Vitreous. Section 12. 2004-2005.* San Francisco, CA: American Academy of Ophthalmology; 2004.
8. Chatterjee S, Tsaloumas MD, Gee H, Lipkin G, Dunne FP. From minimal background diabetic retinopathy to profuse sight-threatening vitreoretinal haemorrhage: management issues in a case of pregestational diabetes and pregnancy. *Diabet Med.* 2003;20(8):683-685.
9. Egan AM, McVicker L, Heerey A, Carmody L, Harney F, Dunne F. Diabetic retinopathy in pregnancy: a population-based study of women with pregestational diabetes. *J Diabetes Res.* 2015;2015:310239. doi: 10.1155/2015/310239.
10. Toda J, Kato S, Sanaka M, Kitano S. The effect of pregnancy on the progression of diabetic retinopathy. *Jpn J Ophthalmol.* 2016;60 (6): 454-458.
11. Pescosolido N, Campagna O, Barbato A. Diabetic retinopathy in pregnancy. A. *Int Ophthalmol.* 2014;34:989-997. doi:10.1007/s10792-014-9906-z
12. Concillado M, Lund-Andersen H, Mathiesen E, Larsen M. Dexamethasone Intravitreal Implant for diabetic macular edema during pregnancy. *Am J Ophthalmol.* 2016;165:7-15.
13. Polizzi S, Mahajan VB. Intravitreal Anti VEGF Injections in Pregnancy. Case Series and Review of Literature . *J Ocul Pharmacol Ther.* 2015;31(10):605-610.

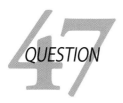

HOW LONG SHOULD I WAIT TO PERFORM CATARACT SURGERY AFTER TREATMENT OF DIABETIC MACULAR EDEMA OR RETINOPATHY?

Linda A. Lam, MD, MBA

A frequent dilemma for cataract surgeons is when to perform surgery in a patient with diabetic retinopathy. Controversy exists regarding cataract surgery and its effects on the development and progression of diabetic macular edema (DME) and diabetic retinopathy. Previous studies reported that cataract surgery in diabetic eyes was complicated by worsening of macular edema and retinopathy with the development of vitreous hemorrhage, anterior segment neovascularization, and worsening visual acuity.[1] Many of these studies were retrospective and included older surgical techniques associated with intra- and extracapsular cataract extraction.[1,2] Recent prospective studies in eyes with relatively low-risk diabetic retinopathy undergoing small-incision phacoemulsification cataract surgery have shown no significant progression of diabetic retinopathy postoperatively compared with that in fellow eyes.[3-6]

In a patient with diabetes who needs cataract surgery, the following should be optimized or treated prior to cataract surgery in order to limit the development and progression of postoperative DME and diabetic retinopathy:

- Degree of glycemic control

- Preoperative severe nonproliferative and proliferative diabetic retinopathy (PDR)

- DME

- Presence of vitreomacular traction (VMT)

Fekrat S, ed. *Curbside Consultation in Retina: 49 Clinical Questions, Second Edition.* (pp 243-246).
© 2019 SLACK Incorporated

Degree of Glycemic Control

Normalizing and stabilizing systemic glucose levels is necessary to reduce the development and progression of diabetic retinopathy after cataract surgery. Poor preoperative glycemic control and poor renal function have been correlated with higher rates of diabetic retinopathy and DME following cataract surgery. Because transient worsening of diabetic retinopathy may occur during the first 6 months of intensive blood glucose management,[7] deferring cataract surgery for at least 6 months is recommended in this scenario.

Preoperative Severe Nonproliferative and Proliferative Diabetic Retinopathy

Patients with severe nonproliferative diabetic retinopathy and PDR may benefit from having panretinal laser photocoagulation (PRP) performed prior to cataract surgery. Cataract surgery can then be delayed for 4 to 6 months afterward to allow the diabetic retinopathy to improve and stabilize. Following PRP, macular edema may subsequently develop or progress. As a result, waiting up to 6 months to perform cataract surgery is reasonable to allow for improvement and sometimes treatment of any secondary DME and regression of any PDR. This may not always be possible as the cataract may be interfere with the delivery of adequate PRP.

Preoperative Diabetic Macular Edema

Preexisting DME is a major contributor to postoperative visual loss in diabetic patients. In eyes with preoperative DME, treatment prior to cataract surgery is recommended as postoperative inflammation can exacerbate edema.[3-6] Postoperative macular edema is common in patients with a history of DME; hence, it is prudent to treat the macular edema prior to cataract extraction.

The most effective treatment options for preoperative DME include anti-vascular endothelial growth factor (anti-VEGF) agents (ie, bevacizumab, ranibizumab, aflibercept). Other options include focal/grid laser, subtenon or intravitreal triamcinolone acetonide, or longer-acting intraocular steroid implants, such as dexamethasone or fluocinolone.

Anti-VEGF agents are the preferred first-line options to reduce DME in an eye with a visually significant cataract. The Diabetic Retinopathy Clinical Research Network explored the effectiveness of the 3 anti-VEGF agents in the treatment of DME.[8] At 2 years, mean visual acuity improved by 12.8, 10, and 12.3 letters in the aflibercept, bevacizumab, and ranibizumab groups, respectively. The differences in visual outcomes among the 3 groups were not statistically significant. While all 3 anti-VEGF agents showed similar rates of improvement in letters gained at year 2 in eyes with initial good baseline vision (20/32 to 20/40), aflibercept showed a statistically significant improvement of visual outcomes in eyes with worse pretreatment vision (worse than 20/50) compared to bevacizumab. No advantage of aflibercept over ranibizumab was found at year 2, while aflibercept remained superior to bevacizumab.

In phakic eyes with DME with a view of the macula, my regimen is to initially start with anti-VEGF therapy for several injections prior to possible focal/grid laser or steroid, if the DME is recalcitrant. The choice of anti-VEGF agent is often dictated by the initial presenting visual acuity and the severity of DME, with aflibercept used more frequently in eyes with severe DME and worse vision. However, given that the visual acuity may be worse due to a cataract that is present, the central retinal thickness plays a more influential role in anti-VEGF drug selection in these eyes with visually significant cataracts. Eyes with worse central retinal thickness (eg, over 400 μm) are more likely to be treated with intravitreal aflibercept.

If the view is sufficient, then fluorescein angiography (FA) can delineate areas of leakage to guide focal/grid laser treatment. If significant DME remains following multiple anti-VEGF treatments or focal/grid laser, intravitreal (or subtenon) triamcinolone can be used to reduce the macular edema. However, steroid treatment may hasten cataract progression and may induce steroid-related intraocular pressure elevation. My preference is to administer intravitreal anti-VEGF injection(s) as first-line treatment followed by FA-guided focal/grid laser to treat DME prior to cataract surgery for an eye with an adequate view of the macula. Cataract surgery should then be delayed 4 to 6 months to allow for improvement of the macular edema.

Recent studies have shown that adjuvant intravitreal anti-VEGF treatment or triamcinolone at the time of cataract surgery may improve macular edema in the short term, up to 6 months.[9] However, long-term data is lacking to support the role of intraoperative adjuvant therapy at this time in the management of preoperative DME.

Eyes without preoperative DME that then develop DME postoperatively usually experience resolution of the edema within the first postoperative year after cataract surgery.[10] Postoperative macular edema therapy should be tailored to whether the edema is related to the Irvine-Gass Syndrome or DME which may be differentiated on FA. If the macular edema shows petaloid leakage (cystoid macular edema) with a hot disc (disc leakage) on FA, then the edema is most likely due to Irvine-Gass Syndrome, and as such, topical anti-inflammatory agents such as topical steroids and topical non-steroidal anti-inflammatory agents are advised as first-line therapy. However, if the FA shows focal leakage from microaneurysms and/or diffuse leakage of diabetic origin, a combination of anti-VEGF treatment and focal/grid laser is recommended. In recalcitrant postoperative macular edema, I also consider intravitreal preservative-free triamcinolone in addition to anti-VEGF agents.[11]

Presence of Vitreomacular Traction

Optical coherence tomography (OCT) can be used to assess the degree of macular edema and evaluate the treatment effect. OCT may reveal the presence of coexisting pathology such as VMT or posterior hyaloidal traction, which may contribute to persistent DME, despite treatment. If significant VMT is present, then vitrectomy may be needed to eliminate the tractional forces contributing to the edema.

If any lens opacity precludes a clear view of the macula for vitreous surgery, then consider either performing cataract surgery prior to vitrectomy or performing both surgeries at the same time. Some retinal surgeons prefer to have the cataract removed first to allow for any associated corneal edema to subside in order to optimize the intraoperative view of the macula.

If the cataract is not severe and the view of the macula is clear enough to allow vitrectomy, I prefer to perform vitrectomy to relieve the VMT and reduce as much of the macular edema as possible prior to cataract surgery. The presence of the macular edema may influence intraocular lens calculations. Allowing the macular edema to resolve prior to cataract surgery would result in a more accurate axial length calculation and consequently, a more appropriate intraocular lens selection. It is possible that intravitreal pharmacotherapeutic agents may have a shorter half-life in some vitrectomized eyes.[12-15]

Summary

Recent data demonstrate that the progression of diabetic retinopathy is not significantly affected by small-incision cataract surgery. However, it is important to treat any preoperative diabetic retinopathy and DME and then allow up to 6 months for improvement and stabilization prior to elective cataract surgery. Key factors such as glycemic control, presence of untreated severe nonproliferative or PDR, DME, and any coexistent VMT need to be addressed prior to proceeding with cataract surgery.

References

1. Mittra RA, Borrillo JL, Dev S. et al. Retinopathy progression and visual outcomes after phacoemulsification in patients with diabetes mellitus. *Arch Ophthalmol.* 2000;118:912-917.
2. Dowler, JG, Sehmi KS, Hykin PG, et al. The natural history of macular edema after cataract surgery in diabetes. *Ophthalmology.* 1999;106:663-668.
3. Romero-Aroca P, Fernández-Ballarat J, Almena-Garcia M, Méndez-Marín I, Salvat-Serra M, Buil-Calvo JA. Nonproliferative diabetic retinopathy and macular edema progression after phacoemulsification: prospective study. *J Cataract Refract Surg.* 2006;32(9):1438-1444.
4. Squirrell D, Bhola R, Bush J, Winder S, Talbot JF. A prospective, case-controlled study of the natural history of diabetic retinopathy and maculopathy after uncomplicated phacoemulsification cataract surgery in patients with type 2 diabetics. *Br J Ophthalmol.* 2002;86(5):565-571.
5. Rashid S, Young LH. Progression of diabetic retinopathy and maculopathy after phacoemulsification surgery. *Int Ophthalmol Clin.* 2010;50(1):155-166.
6. Shah AS, Chen SH. Cataract surgery and diabetes. *Curr Opin Ophthalmol.* 2010;21(1):4-9.
7. Diabetes Control and Complications Trial Research Group. Early worsening of diabetic retinopathy in the diabetes control and complications trial. *Arch Ophthalmol.* 1998;116(7):874-886.
8. Wells JA, Glassman AR, Ayala AR, et al. Aflibercept, bevacizumab, or ranibizumab for diabetic macular edema: two year results from a comparative effectiveness randomized clinical trial. *Ophthalmology.* 2016;123(6):1351-1359.
9. Cetlin EN, Yildirim C. Adjuvant treatment modalities to control macular edema in diabetic patients undergoing cataract surgery. *Int Ophthalmol.* 2013;33(5):605-610.
10. Murtha T, Cavallerano J. The management of diabetic eye disease in the setting of cataract surgery. *Curr Opin Ophthalmol.* 2007;18(1):13-18.
11. Grover D, Li TJ, Chong CC. Intravitreal steroids for macular edema in diabetes. *Cochrane Database Syst Rev.* 2008;(1): CD005656.
12. Ahn J, Kim H, Woo SJ, et al. Pharmacokinetics of intravitreally injected Bevacizumab in vitrectomized eyes. *J Ocul Pharmacol Ther.* 2013;29(7):612-618.
13. Ahn, SJ, Ahn J, Park S, et al. Intraocular pharmacokinetics of Ranibizumab in vitrectomized versus nonvitrectomized eyes. *Invest Ophthalmol Vis Sci.* 2014;55(1):567-573.
14. Christoforidis JB, Carlton MM, Wang J, et al. Anatomic and pharmacokinetic properties of intravitreal bevacizumab and ranibizumab after vitrectomy and lensectomy. *Retina.* 2013;33(5):946-952.
15. Papastefanou, V. Pharmacokinetics of anti-VEGF and steroid agents in vitrectomized eyes with diabetic macular edema. *Acta Ophthalmol.* 2015;93. doi: 10.1111/j.1755-3768.2015.0127.

QUESTION 48

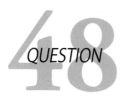

I Saw Some Retinal Neovascularization but My Patient Does Not Have Diabetes, so What Else Can It Be?

Brian E. Goldhagen, MD

While diabetes is certainly the most common cause of retinal neovascularization, it is also important to consider other causes when evaluating a patient, particularly when the clinical picture does not fit. Retinal neovascularization occurs when new abnormal blood vessels proliferate from preexisting retinal vessels due to a pro-angiogenic stimulus, the source of which is often ischemia. The detection and accurate diagnosis of this retinal finding is imperative. Untreated retinal neovascularization has the potential to lead to devastating ocular complications, including tractional retinal detachment and neovascular glaucoma due to associated anterior segment neovascularization, which can result in irreversible vision loss. Understanding the underlying cause for the neovascularization is not only important in attempting to prevent these ocular complications, but also in the management or possibly even the diagnosis of an underlying systemic condition and thus the protection of the fellow eye. Perhaps the patient actually does have diabetes and it simply is not diagnosed yet.

There is a rather large differential diagnosis for retinal neovascularization, which may seem overwhelming at first (Table 48-1).[1] When I see retinal neovascularization, I begin by attempting to further assess and describe what it is that I am seeing on exam. What does the neovascularization look like and where is it located? Is it located peripherally or closer to the posterior pole, perhaps even involving the optic nerve? I also find it helpful to remember that neovascularization is almost never an isolated ocular exam finding; therefore, I pay particular attention to any other abnormal findings that may be present including their distribution. I also take note of any inflammation or vasculitis that may be present. Finally, I make sure to pay attention to the actual patient presenting before me including the presenting symptoms, age, gender, and any pertinent past medical or family history.

Fekrat S, ed. *Curbside Consultation in Retina: 49 Clinical Questions, Second Edition*. (pp 247-250).
© 2019 SLACK Incorporated

Table 48-1
Causes of Retinal Neovascularization

Neovascularization of the Posterior Pole/Mid-Periphery	Neovascularization of the Retinal Periphery
• Proliferative diabetic retinopathy • Central retinal vein occlusion (CRVO) • Branch retinal vein occlusion (BRVO) • Ocular ischemic syndrome (OIS) • Radiation retinopathy	• Retinopathy of prematurity (ROP) • Familial exudative vitreoretinopathy • Hemoglobinopathies • Hyperviscosity syndromes • Uveitis

I generally try to think of the diseases that cause retinal neovascularization as belonging to 1 of 2 basic groups: those with the neovascularization found at the posterior pole and mid-periphery and those with more peripheral neovascularization. This second group I further subdivide into those with evidence of inflammation or vasculitis and those without.

Retinal Neovascularization at the Posterior Pole and Mid-Periphery

When I see neovascularization and findings closer to the posterior pole, I typically begin thinking of cardiovascular-related ocular diseases including proliferative diabetic retinopathy, CRVO, BRVO, and in some cases, OIS. Although retinal artery occlusion is also related to cardiovascular disease, it rarely manifests with retinal neovascularization, but rather, more commonly with anterior segment neovascularization.

Funduscopic examination in diabetes, vein occlusion, and OIS often include microaneurysms, dot-blot hemorrhages, cotton-wool spots, vascular attenuation, and/or macular edema. Lipid exudates are more commonly seen in diabetic retinopathy, whereas flame hemorrhages are more common in vein occlusions. The laterality of retinal findings is helpful in differentiating these diseases, with diabetic retinopathy typically having bilateral findings as compared to both vein occlusion and OIS, which are usually unilateral.

In distinguishing vein occlusions from OIS, OIS typically presents with hemorrhages located in the mid-periphery and periphery and veins that are described as dilated but not tortuous.[2] Carotid imaging should be ordered in any patient where OIS is suspected. CRVO typically presents with unilateral vision loss in patients over 60 years of age with a known history of hypertension. Atypical presentations should prompt further investigation with particular attention to hypercoagulable states and risk factors for thrombosis, including a review of the patient's medical history, family history, and medications, as well as laboratory studies.

Radiation retinopathy also manifests with posterior findings and may have retinal neovascularization. Ophthalmoscopically, it looks very similar to diabetic retinopathy except that microaneurysms are rarely seen. On further questioning, these patients will typically endorse having a recent history, usually within the past few years, of radiation treatment.

Peripheral Retinal Neovascularization

When the retinal neovascularization and other retinal findings are more peripheral in location, I pay particular attention to evidence of vasculitis or inflammation. If these are not present, I begin thinking about hemoglobinopathies, ROP, familial exudative vitreoretinopathy (FEVR), and hyperviscosity syndromes. Conditions resulting from exogenous embolization, such as talc retinopathy, may also be considered when multiple small emboli are present. Such findings should prompt further questioning about intravenous drug abuse.

The hemoglobinopathies include sickle cell trait (AS), sickle cell disease (SS), sickle cell hemoglobin C disease (SC), hemoglobin C trait (AC), and sickle beta thalassemia (Sβthal), of which SC and Sβthal are the most likely to have retinal disease.[3] Often, patients are unaware that they are carriers when they do not have systemic manifestations, and as such, a discussion about lab work to confirm the diagnosis as well as possible genetic counseling may be indicated. Like other peripheral causes of retinal neovascularization, dot-blot hemorrhages are an uncommon finding. Instead, oval salmon patch hemorrhages, glistening iridescent spots, and hyperpigmented black sunbursts are typically seen. The neovascularization has a sea fan appearance and is typically seen at the border of perfused and nonperfused retina.

While ROP and FEVR look rather distinct from the other retinal diseases, and typically initially present in younger patients, they look quite similar to one another.[4] Funduscopic features include bilateral peripheral nonperfusion with adjacent arteriovenous shunts, microaneurysms, and temporal macular dragging. The fundamental difference between these 2 entities lies in the history; patients with FEVR often have a family history of similar retinal findings and are typically born full-term without a history of supplemental oxygen. Although incontinentia pigmenti is also on the differential for retinal neovascularization in younger individuals, it is typically easily distinguishable based on its accompanying characteristic skin and nervous system abnormalities.

Hyperviscosity syndromes may also manifest with retinal neovascularization, the most common of which is Waldenstrom macroglobulinemia. Funduscopically, this looks similar to bilateral CRVO; however, the presence of serous retinal detachments without significant intraretinal fluid should raise suspicion for this as the causative etiology. That being said, patients with Waldenstrom macroglobulinemia rarely initially present with ocular manifestations, and a thorough review of the patient's medical history and review of systems are useful clues to establishing the diagnosis. Chronic myeloid leukemia is another hyperviscosity syndrome that may lead to peripheral retinal neovascularization.

Retinal Neovascularization With Inflammation/Vasculitis

When I see neovascularization present in a patient with ocular inflammation or vasculitis, other types of eye conditions come to mind. Intermediate uveitis is typically on the top of my differential, particularly pars planitis and sarcoidosis-related uveitis. Pars planitis is an idiopathic type of intermediate uveitis characterized by snowballs and snowbanks; however, these findings may be present in sarcoidosis as well. It is along the inferior snowbanks that retinal neovascularization, with the potential to lead to vitreous hemorrhage or retinal detachment, is most commonly seen. Both pars planitis and sarcoidosis typically have bilateral findings and may also demonstrate macular edema and periphlebitis. The periphlebitis classically appears like candle wax drippings in sarcoidosis. Sarcoidosis may also present as a panuveitis with chorioretinal lesions and/or keratic precipitates. Obtaining a chest X-ray or blood test for angiotensin-converting enzyme may aid in the diagnosis. Chronic retinal vasculitis of any etiology may also lead to retinal neovascularization.

When periphlebitis is present with peripheral neovascularization, but without evidence of intermediate uveitis, I would start considering other conditions, including Eales' disease. This idiopathic occlusive perivasculitis most commonly affects otherwise healthy young men and features peripheral inflammatory BRVOs and venous sheathing.[5] Patients with Eales' disease classically present with an acute onset of unilateral blurred vision and floaters secondary to vitreous hemorrhage from peripheral neovascularization. Eales' disease is a diagnosis of exclusion, and other causes of vasocclusive disease should first be considered. These include those diseases with peripheral neovascularization that also have systemic findings, including lupus, Takayasu arteritis (aortic arch syndrome), Susac syndrome, and syphilis.

What If You Are Still Unsure About What Is Causing the Retinal Neovascularization?

If I am still uncertain as to the cause of the retinal neovascularization after careful history taking and a complete ocular examination, I usually will attempt to better understand the retinal vasculature through fluorescein angiography. Additional clues may be elucidated through a full physical exam as well as lab work directed by pertinent findings. Involving the patient's internist may also be useful, especially because understanding the reason for the neovascularization may be important in the management or possibly even the diagnosis of an underlying systemic condition.

References

1. Jampol LM, Ebroon DA, Goldbaum MH. Peripheral proliferative retinopathies: an update on angiogenesis, etiologies and management. *Surv Ophthalmol.* 1994;38(6):519-540.
2. Brown GC, Magargal LE. The ocular ischemic syndrome. Clinical, fluorescein angiographic and carotid angiographic features. *Int Ophthalmol.* 1988;11(4):239-251.
3. Goldberg MF. Natural history of untreated proliferative sickle retinopathy. *Arch Ophthalmol.* 1971;85(4):428-437.
4. Canny CL, Oliver GL. Fluorescein angiographic findings in familial exudative vitreoretinopathy. *Arch Ophthalmol.* 1976;94(7):1114-1120.
5. Biswas J, Sharma T, Gopal L, Madhavan HN, Sulochana KN, Ramakrishnan S. Eales disease—an update. *Surv Ophthalmol.* 2002;47(3):197-214.

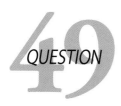

WHEN SHOULD I CONSIDER ANTI-VASCULAR ENDOTHELIAL GROWTH FACTOR TREATMENT FOR RETINOPATHY OF PREMATURITY?

Yoshihiro Yonekawa, MD
Kimberly A. Drenser, MD, PhD

Retinopathy of prematurity (ROP) is a vascular endothelial growth factor (VEGF)–driven disease, so why not treat all infants using anti-VEGF agents? It makes sense physiologically, and it fits into the current drift of treating seemingly every retinal or choroidal vasculopathy with local VEGF suppression. Unfortunately, it's much more complex for ROP, and there are several key factors to consider that we will outline. But first, we will preface by mentioning that there is no consensus on laser vs anti-VEGF treatment for ROP. Some practitioners use only laser, some use only anti-VEGF, while most use a thoughtfully titrated combination of the 2, and end up somewhere along the spectrum based on patient population, neonatal intensive care unit capabilities, access to resources, and surgeon preference. The following are our personal preferences at the time of writing, which may also evolve as we accumulate more evidence.

ROP occurs in 2 phases. In the vaso-obliterative phase, high oxygen tension attenuates the retinal vasculature and halts its growth from the optic disc towards the peripheral retina. In the subsequent vasoproliferative phase, arteriovenous shunting occurs at the vascular-avascular junction where retinal fibrovascular proliferation occurs in response to the ischemic peripheral retina. One of the key cytokines during this vasoproliferative phase is indeed VEGF, and suppressing VEGF during this phase does promote ROP regression.

Off-label use of anti-VEGF agents for ROP is increasing throughout the world since its first descriptions a decade ago.[1] Avastin (bevacizumab) is currently the most commonly used, and most practitioners use half of the adult dose (0.625 mg), although the optimal dose has not yet been determined. We prefer using Lucentis (ranibizumab) if possible, because it does not suppress systemic circulating VEGF as much (though it is unknown if this is a clinically meaningful benefit). The main drawbacks of ranibizumab are that it is difficult to access for ROP because it is not a

Fekrat S, ed. *Curbside Consultation in Retina: 49 Clinical Questions, Second Edition.* (pp 251-253).
© 2019 SLACK Incorporated

US Food and Drug Administration–approved indication, and that recurrence of plus disease and neovascularization are more common than with bevacizumab, and the recurrences tend to occur sooner.

There are many benefits of anti-VEGF monotherapy. First, it's easy to administer from a logistic, technical, and economic (if using bevacizumab) standpoint. A bedside injection under local anesthesia takes only a few moments; the infant does not have to undergo general anesthesia that may have associated systemic risk (as a cohort, these are arguably the highest risk patients in our field). Additionally, bevacizumab is widely available and cheap; an intravitreal injection is technically much easier to perform than thorough laser, and injections are possible, even through media opacities. Studies have also shown that the rates of pathologic myopia are less compared to eyes that have been lasered, and most intriguingly, the retinal vasculature can continue to grow into the periphery after anti-VEGF treatment.[2,3] Visual fields are therefore more preserved compared to ablative laser treatment.

There are, however, potential drawbacks of anti-VEGF treatment. Organogenesis is still occurring in premature infants, and VEGF is known to play a key role in development of the lungs, kidneys, brain, etc. Intravitreally injected anti-VEGF agents, especially bevacizumab, have been shown to enter the systemic circulation and suppress VEGF levels throughout the body. Thankfully no studies to date have shown whether this temporary suppression of systemic VEGF has any clinical effects. Two small retrospective studies placed the issue on the radar by suggesting an effect on neurodevelopment, but the studies are far from being definitive.[4] This issue will be very hard to tease out because these infants often have severe systemic comorbidities that cause multiple chronic diseases including those that affect neurodevelopment.

Another downside of anti-VEGF treatment is the unpredictable recurrences that may sometimes occur many months after the injection.[5] This unpredictability makes the follow-up schedule challenging. The children also become more difficult to examine in clinic as they get older. It has been suggested that infants be followed weekly until a postmenstrual age of 72 weeks. With laser treatment, the course of disease is very predictable, and we have a defined endpoint of when to stop screening, and late recurrences are not an issue. Therefore, if an infant does not fully vascularize with anti-VEGF treatment, many practitioners will laser the residual avascular retina.

The last downside of anti-VEGF treatment is the higher potential for crunching of the fibrotic component of the fibrovascular membranes, which can lead to progressive tractional retinal detachment. We have recently shown that these retinal detachments can have unique configurations that can be relatively difficult to operate on.[6] As the infants approach term, the VEGF levels decrease in the eye, and there is an endogenous rise in transforming growth factor-beta (TGF-β). When VEGF is artificially suppressed pharmacologically, TGF-β rises also. As TGF-β is a profibrotic cytokine, the surges from both endogenous and pharmacologic routes may lead to crunching of the fibrovascular membranes and associated posterior hyaloid. This appears to occur more commonly in eyes with aggressive posterior-ROP, or if the injection takes place relatively later. If injected timely at the first signs of Type I ROP, we feel that this phenomenon may be avoidable.

As there are benefits and downsides to both laser and anti-VEGF treatment, the risks and benefits need to be weighed carefully for each individual patient. We do not recommend a one-size-fits-all paradigm for ROP treatment, because there are many variables at play as outlined previously. Please note that every ROP-treating physician has a management algorithm that works best for them and their patients. That being said, this is how the authors' groups currently recommend using anti-VEGF agents given the presently available data (again, every patient is different, so this is a flexible guideline).

First, anti-VEGF treatment is recommended if laser photocoagulation is not available. Most of the ROP burden is now occurring in middle-income nations, and many hospitals still do not have access to indirect laser systems. Anti-VEGF treatment is certainly better than no treatment.

Second, we consider anti-VEGF treatment if the fovea is not vascularized, and laser treatment would require lasering the fovea. Anti-VEGF treatment usually allows the vasculature to grow through the macula. However, we have shown that the macula does develop to a surprising degree after laser treatment, so you should not be faulted if the presumed area of the fovea needs to be lasered.

Third, anti-VEGF agents work well if there are media opacities that prevent adequate laser application. This includes an intensely dilated tunica vasculosa lentis and neovascularization, and vitreous hemorrhage. However, if there is any suspicion for tractional membranes or retinal detachment, or if the vitreous hemorrhage is too dense for an accurate examination, we would proceed with pars plicata vitrectomy.

Fourth, anti-VEGF is indicated if the infant cannot medically tolerate laser photocoagulation. The sickest infants may not be able to tolerate general anesthesia and/or may become hemodynamically unstable with laser application. In these instances, which are not rare in this patient population, the quick intravitreal injection may be the best option. The least stable infants may be a poor choice for anti-VEGF treatment, however, as they theoretically have the greatest risk from systemic suppression of circulating VEGF. In particular, the risk of worsening their bronchopulmonary dysplasia should be discussed with the neonatologist and parents prior to any treatment.

Fifth, we consider anti-VEGF treatment only if reliable follow-up is possible. If the family cannot commit to close observation for any reason, laser photocoagulation is preferred.

Finally, we always present the option of laser vs anti-VEGF to the parents, and if the parents prefer anti-VEGF treatment after a balanced informed consent process that discusses all of the points aforementioned, we would offer anti-VEGF monotherapy as a starting point. It is important to discuss what off-label means and check with your malpractice insurance to ensure coverage for anti-VEGF use in infants.

For all other patients, which are the majority, we prefer to treat with laser photocoagulation, due to its proven efficacy, predictable response, and lack of effect on systemic VEGF. Having the peripheral retina lasered makes vitrectomy easier should it become necessary and treats avascular retina which presents a risk for future retinal tears and detachment. Again, these are our personal preferences, and there is no one correct answer at the current time.

There is a lot to learn about anti-VEGF treatment for infants with ROP, and we hope that ongoing clinical trials will provide better evidence.[7] For the time being, both laser photocoagulation and anti-VEGF agents play important roles in the treatment of infants with ROP, and it is up to the practitioner to carefully evaluate individual infants to determine the best management plan to maximize outcomes and minimize complications for this vulnerable patient population.

References

1. Quiroz-Mercado H, Martinez-Castellanos MA, Hernandez-Rojas ML, et al. Antiangiogenic therapy with intravitreal bevacizumab for retinopathy of prematurity. *Retina*. 2008;28(Suppl):S19-25.
2. Lepore D, Quinn GE, Molle F, et al. Intravitreal bevacizumab versus laser treatment in type 1 retinopathy of prematurity: report on fluorescein angiographic findings. *Ophthalmology*. 2014;121(11):2212-2219.
3. Geloneck MM, Chuang AZ, Clark WL, et al. Refractive outcomes following bevacizumab monotherapy compared with conventional laser treatment: a randomized clinical trial. *JAMA Ophthalmol*. 2014;132(11):1327-1333.
4. Morin J, Luu TM, Superstein R, et al. Neurodevelopmental outcomes following bevacizumab injections for retinopathy of prematurity. *Pediatrics*. 2016;137(4):e20153218.
5. Wong RK, Hubschman S, Tsui I. Reactivation of retinopathy of prematurity after ranibizumab treatment. *Retina*. 2015;35(4):675-680.
6. Yonekawa Y, Wu WC, Nitulescu CE, et al. Progressive retinal detachment in infants with retinopathy of prematurity treated with intravitreal bevacizumab or ranibizumab. *Retina*. 2018;38(6):1079-1083.
7. ClinicalTrials.gov. RAINBOW study: ranibizumab compared with laser therapy for the treatment of infants born prematurely with retinopathy of prematurity. https://clinicaltrials.gov/ct2/show/NCT02375971. Updated March 6, 2018. Accessed April 30, 2018.

FINANCIAL DISCLOSURES

Dr. Jackson Abou Chehade has no financial or proprietary interest in the materials presented herein.

Dr. Ron A. Adelman has no financial or proprietary interest in the materials presented herein.

Dr. A. Yasin Alibhai has no financial or proprietary interest in the materials presented herein.

Dr. Michael T. Andreoli has no financial or proprietary interest in the materials presented herein.

Dr. Sophie J. Bakri has no financial or proprietary interest in the materials presented herein.

Dr. Alexander Barash has no financial or proprietary interest in the materials presented herein.

Dr. Caroline R. Baumal has no financial or proprietary interest in the materials presented herein.

Dr. Daniel G. Cherfan has no financial or proprietary interest in the materials presented herein.

Dr. Michael N. Cohen has no financial or proprietary interest in the materials presented herein.

Dr. Daniel Connors has no financial or proprietary interest in the materials presented herein.

Dr. Felipe F. Conti has no financial or proprietary interest in the materials presented herein.

Dr. Alessa Crossan has no financial or proprietary interest in the materials presented herein.

Cathy DiBernardo is a paid image grader for Aura Biosciences, Inc.

Dr. Diana V. Do has no financial or proprietary interest in the materials presented herein.

Dr. Bernard H. Doft has no financial or proprietary interest in the materials presented herein.

Dr. Mallika Doss has no financial or proprietary interest in the materials presented herein.

Dr. Kimberly A. Drenser has ownership interest in FocusROP and equity in Phoenix.

Dr. Justis P. Ehlers is a consultant for Zeiss, Leica, Alcon, Thrombogenics, Regeneron, Aerpio, Genetech, Roche, Allergan, and Alimera; and receives research support from Alcon, Thrombogenics, Regeneron, Genetech, Aerpio, and Boerhinger-Ingelheim.

Dr. Dean Eliott has no financial or proprietary interest in the materials presented herein.

Dr. Nicholas Farber has no financial or proprietary interest in the materials presented herein.

Dr. Amani A. Fawzi has no financial or proprietary interest in the materials presented herein.

Dr. Sharon Fekrat receives patent royalties from Alcon and is a consultant for Regeneron.

Dr. Avni P. Finn has no financial or proprietary interest in the materials presented herein.

Dr. Harry W. Flynn, Jr. received support from the NIH Center Core Grant P30EY014801 and received an Unrestricted Grant from Research to Prevent Blindness.

Dr. Jose Mauricio Botto Garcia has no financial or proprietary interest in the materials presented herein.

Dr. Seema Garg has no financial or proprietary interest in the materials presented herein.

Dr. Karen M. Gehrs has no financial or proprietary interest in the materials presented herein.

Dr. Ronald C. Gentile receives grants and/or research support from Genetech, Regeneron, Sirion Therapeutics, National Institutes of Health, University of Wisconsin, Allergan, Alcon, OHR Pharmaceuticals, and DRCRnet.

Dr. Marina Gilca has no financial or proprietary interest in the materials presented herein.

Dr. Brian E. Goldhagen has no financial or proprietary interest in the materials presented herein.

Dr. Margaret A. Greven is a consultant for Alimera Sciences.

Dr. Dilraj S. Grewal is a consultant for Allergan and Alimera Sciences.

Dr. Paul Hahn is a consultant for Second Sight Medical Products.

Dr. Andrew M. Hendrick is a consultant for Clearside Biomedical.

Dr. Odette Margit Houghton has no financial or proprietary interest in the materials presented herein.

Dr. Thomas Hwang has no financial or proprietary interest in the materials presented herein.

Dr. Alessandro Iannaccone receives research funding from Applied Genetic Technologies Corp (AGTC) and is a consultant for Ionis Pharmaceuticals.

Dr. Raymond Iezzi has no financial or proprietary interest in the materials presented herein.

Dr. Michael S. Ip is a consultant for Omeros, Thrombogenics, Genetech, Quark, Boehringer, Ingelheim, Allergan, Alimera, and Allergo.

Dr. Yali Jia has received a research grant and patent royalty from Optovue Inc.

Dr. Scott Ketner has not disclosed any relevant financial disclosures.

Dr. Judy E. Kim is a consultant for Alimera Science, Genentech, and Notal Vision.

Ryan S. Kim has no financial or proprietary interest in the materials presented herein.

Dr. Todd R. Klesert has no financial or proprietary interest in the materials presented herein.

Dr. Linda A. Lam has no financial or proprietary interest in the materials presented herein.

Dr. Jeremy A. Lavine has no financial or proprietary interest in the materials presented herein.

Dr. Jennifer I. Lim has no financial or proprietary interest in the materials presented herein.

Dr. Phoebe Lin is on the advisory boards for Mallinckrodt and Clearside.

Dr. T. Y. Alvin Liu has no financial or proprietary interest in the materials presented herein.

Dr. Tamer H. Mahmoud has no financial or proprietary interest in the materials presented herein.

Dr. Joseph N. Martel has no financial or proprietary interest in the materials presented herein.

Dr. Pauline T. Merrill has no financial or proprietary interest in the materials presented herein.

Dr. Catherine B. Meyerle has no financial or proprietary interest in the materials presented herein.

Dr. William F. Mieler has no financial or proprietary interest in the materials presented herein.

Dr. Prithvi Mruthyunjaya is a consultant for Optos, Castle Biosciences Inc, and SPARK Therapeutics.

Dr. Lisa C. Olmos de Koo is on the scientific advisory board for Alcon Surgical R+D, Science Based Health.

Dr. Kaivon Pakzad-Vaezi has no financial or proprietary interest in the materials presented herein.

Dr. Amar Patel has no financial or proprietary interest in the materials presented herein.

Dr. Kathryn L. Pepple has no financial or proprietary interest in the materials presented herein.

Dr. Sean M. Platt has no financial or proprietary interest in the materials presented herein.

Dr. Matthew A. Powers has no financial or proprietary interest in the materials presented herein.

Dr. Franco M. Recchia receives research support from Roche/Genetech and Regeneron.

Dr. Nidhi Relhan Batra has no financial or proprietary interest in the materials presented herein.

Dr. Kourous A. Rezaei is a consultant for Alcon Laboratories.

Dr. Philipp Roberts has no financial or proprietary interest in the materials presented herein.

Dr. Philip J. Rosenfeld receives research support from Carl Zeiss Meditec, Genentech, and Tyrogenex; is a consultant for Achillion Pharmaceuticals, Acucela, Boehringer-Ingelheim, Carl Zeiss Meditec, Cell Cure Neurosciences, Chengdu Kanghong Biotech, Ocunexus Therapeutics, Genentech, Healios K.K, Hemera Biosciences, F. Hoffmann-La Roche Ltd., Isarna Pharmaceuticals, Lin Bioscience, MacRegen Inc, NGM Biopharmaceuticals, Ocunexus, Ocudyne, Tyrogenex, and Unity Biotechnology; and has equity interest in Apellis, Digisight, and Ocudyne.

Dr. SriniVas R. Sadda is a consultant for ThromboGenics.

Dr. Amy C. Schefler has no financial or proprietary interest in the materials presented herein.

Dr. Stephen G. Schwartz, within the past 3 years, has received funding outside the submitted work from Alimera and Welch Allyn; this work was partially supported by NIH Center Core Grant P30EY014801 and an Unrestricted Grant from Research to Prevent Blindness to the University of Miami.

Dr. Steven D. Schwartz has not disclosed any relevant financial disclosures.

Dr. Ingrid U. Scott has no financial or proprietary interest in the materials presented herein.

Dr. Michael I. Seider has no financial or proprietary interest in the materials presented herein.

Dr. Gaurav K. Shah is a consultant for Allergan, Bausch + Lomb, Johnson & Johnson, QLT Ophthalmics Inc, and Regeneron.

Dr. Sumit Sharma has no financial or proprietary interest in the materials presented herein.

Dr. Fabiana Q. Silva has no financial or proprietary interest in the materials presented herein.

Dr. Rishi P. Singh us a consultant for Regeneron, Genentech, Zeiss, and Optos; and receives grant support from Regeneron, Roche, Alcon, and Apellis.

Dr. Richard F. Spaide is a consultant for Topcon Medical Systems.

Dr. Sunil K. Srivastava has no financial or proprietary interest in the materials presented herein.

Dr. James A. Stefater has no financial or proprietary interest in the materials presented herein.

Dr. Akshay Thomas has no financial or proprietary interest in the materials presented herein.

Dr. Arthi Venkat has no financial or proprietary interest in the materials presented herein.

Dr. Elizabeth Verner-Cole has no financial or proprietary interest in the materials presented herein.

Dr. Nadia K. Waheed is a consultant for Regeneron, Genetech, Janssen and Janessen, Optovue, and Nidek; and receives research support from Carl Zeiss Meditec.

Dr. Scott D. Walter receives research support from Heed Ophthalmic Foundation, ASCRS Foundation, and Research to Prevent Blindness.

Dr. Charles C. Wykoff has no financial or proprietary interest in the materials presented herein.

Dr. Glenn Yiu has no financial or proprietary interest in the materials presented herein.

Dr. Yoshihiro Yonekawa has no financial or proprietary interest in the materials presented herein.

Index